toxins

Botulinum toxin in aesthetic medicine: injection protocols and complication management

Jani van Loghem, MD PhD

UMA academy

CRC Press
Taylor & Francis Group
Boca Raton London New York

CRC Press is an imprint of the
Taylor & Francis Group, an **informa** business

Know what can go wrong.
Know what can go right.
Know why something works, and when it won't.
Know the difference between good and great.
Know what a patient wants, and what they need.
Know when to push on. Know when to stop.
Know why you're being cautious, or brave.
Know what you don't know.
Know more than the products in your dispensary.
Know more than the treatments you offer,
or the tools you use to deliver them.
Know how to express who your patient wants to be.

knowledge is beautiful

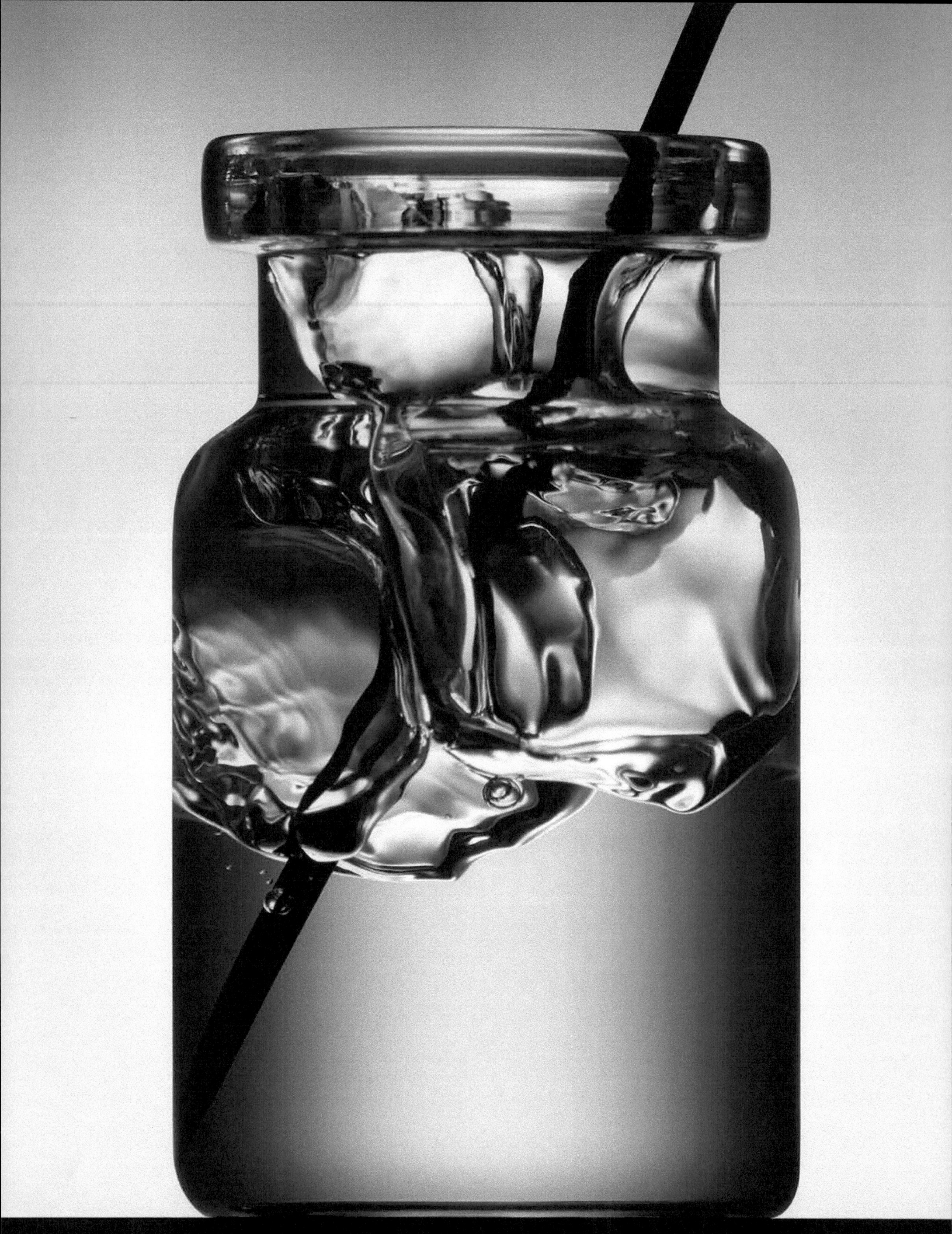

Cover design by UMA
Text design by Rosa Koolhoven and Eszter Takács /Eszter Design
Photography by Bart Oomes and Casper van der Linde
Videos by Casper van der Linde

This edition published 2023
by CRC Press
6000 Broken Sound Parkway NW, Suite 300, Boca Raton, FL 33487-2742

and by CRC Press
4 Park Square, Milton Park, Abingdon, Oxon, OX14 4RN

CRC Press is an imprint of Taylor & Francis Group, LLC

Library of Congress Cataloging-in-Publication Data

ISBN: 978-1-032-44053-8 (hbk)
ISBN: 978-1-032-44054-5 (pbk)
ISBN: 978-1-003-37018-5 (ebk)

DOI: 10.1201/9781003370185

Typeset in Optima
by KnowledgeWorks Global Ltd.

let's talk botulinum toxin

Injection Protocols and Complication Management

table of contents

table of contents

introduction

Dear colleagues,

As the field of aesthetic medicine grows, more and more aesthetic physicians seek structured education in order to optimize the safety and quality of the treatments they offer. I enjoy being a trainer and educator as much as I enjoy treating my patients and feel an obligation to share my experience and practical tips with my fellow aesthetic physicians. I have therefore started UMA Academy as a basis for quality aesthetic education, focusing predominantly on hands-on training.

Protocols
As protocols and standardized treatments play an increasingly important part in the development of aesthetic medicine as a medical field, various consensus papers have been published to provide physicians with standard protocols for botulinum toxin injection therapy. The protocols described here have been developed using consensus recommendations from a number of consensus groups and various publications published by the Dutch Society of Aesthetic Medicine, the Deutsche Gesellschaft für Dermatologie, The European Academy of Dermatology and Venereology, The American Society for Dermatologic Surgery, The American Academy of Otolaryngology, Head and Neck Surgery, and the American Academy of Cosmetic Surgery. For the final recommendations in these standard protocols, we, the physicians of UMA Institute, have adjusted the injection patterns and doses slightly to optimize efficacy, while minimizing risks of side effects.

eBook
This practical book is meant for quick review during day-to-day practice in aesthetic medicine. We have included limited background information about botulinum toxin: the history, mechanism of action, the different available products with similarities and differences, reconstitution, patient consultation, documentation and photography, physical examination, marking and preparing for injection. More emphasis is placed on practical uses of botulinum toxin such as injection patterns, relevant anatomy and avoiding and treating complications.

The use of Bocouture® (Xeomin®)
In our clinic, we use IncobotulinumtoxinA (Bocouture®/ Xeomin®; Merz Aesthetics GmbH, Frankfurt, Germany). The reason for this choice is that we do not introduce an unnecessary risk of immunogenicity to our patients as this product is free from complexing proteins. For patients who are very keen on having natural results, we have introduced a new way of treating with this product which uses only half the recommended doses shown in the protocols in this book. Of course, this reduces duration, so we retreat these patients every 2-3 months instead of every 4 months. This provides a non-blocked, more subtle refreshed and relaxed result and is typically what many of our patients want nowadays. Bocouture®/ Xeomin® is the only toxin that can be used with such short treatment intervals. Other patients prefer a more blocked effect with very long duration. For these individuals, the recommended dose may be increased up to 5 times, keeping in mind that the risk of side effects increases. In this book we also discuss OnabotulinumtoxinA (Vistabel®/ Botox®; Allergan Inc., Irvine, CA, USA) and AbobotulinumtoxinA (Azzalure®/ Dysport®; Ipsen, Paris, France) and provide recommended doses and injection schemes.

We hope this book will be of value to you, your clinic and your patients. Please let us know if you have any ideas for improvement as we would love to hear from you.

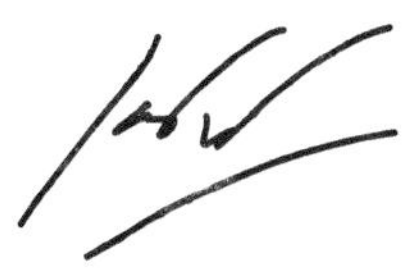

Jani van Loghem, MD PhD
Founder UMA Institute
academy@uma-institute.com

01
general background

introduction

Apart from theoretical and practical knowhow, a broad understanding of all aesthetic treatment methods is a requirement for the practitioner to safely offer botulinum toxin treatment and to assess whether this treatment is the first choice for the patient requesting botulinum toxin therapy.

Besides a medical degree, a well-structured training program that assesses both the theoretical and practical skills of the practitioner is a prerequisite for the botulinum toxin injector.

general

1.1 History of botulinum toxin

In 1817, Dr. Justinus Kerner described the disease botulism, a serious form of food poisoning, resulting in symmetric overall muscle paralysis leading to death. The likely cause of this condition in the publication of Kerner was identified as spoiled sausages. Kerner concluded from his research that a diluted form of the poison could be used in the treatment of patients with muscular hyper-motility disorders. Further research on botulism led to the isolation of *Clostridium Botulinum* which is a large, spore-forming, anaerobic bacterium. This was followed by the isolation of botulinum toxin type A and subsequent clinical testing and application in hyperkinetic disorders, including blepharospasm and strabismus. In 1992, the Canadian couple Jean (ophthalmologist) and Alistair (dermatologist) Carruthers published the first scientific study about botulinum toxin for the aesthetic treatment of the glabella. Patients that were treated for blepharo-spasm showed a reduction of dynamic wrinkles. This observation had a huge impact on the world of aesthetic medicine and botulinum toxin is now the most important instrument of many aesthetic practitioners.

1.2 Mechanism of action

The protein botulinum toxin is a double chain poly-peptide molecule that is produced by the bacterium *Clostridium Botulinum*. It consists of a light chain (50kD) and a heavy chain (100 kD). After injection, the botulinum toxin protein binds with the heavy chain to presynaptic receptor SV1 and endocytosis occurs. The heavy chain forms a pore in the membrane of the endocytosis vacuole so that the short-chain can be released into the cytoplasm, and exert its pharmacological effect. Seven different variants are known (type A to G), of which type A is the most potent. The mechanism of action of all variants is based on blocking the signal from the neuronal axon to the neuromuscular junction by preventing fusion of the acetylcholine neurotransmitter vacuoles with the presynaptic membrane. The different variants of botulinum toxin target a different presynaptic protein. Botulinum toxin type A selectively targets SNAP-25, part of the SNARE complex and one of the intracellular presynaptic proteins that is essential for fusing acetyl choline vacuoles with the presynaptic membrane after the electric stimulus reaches the end of the axon.
With SNAP-25 cleaved by the light chain, the SNARE complex doesn't work, the acetyl choline vacuole cannot fuse, and therefore the neurotransmitter will remain intracellular instead of reaching the synapse. The motor neuron is then blocked for approximately 3-4 months.

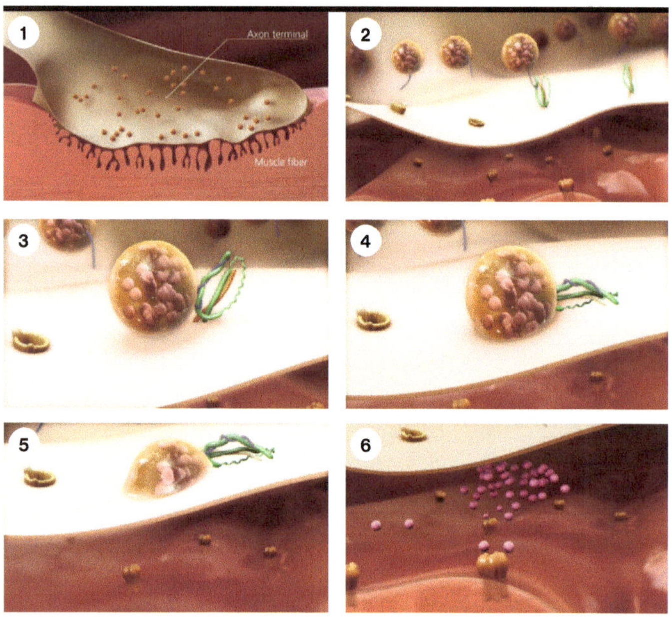

Images kindly provided by Merz Aesthetics

Figure 1
Mechanism of action of botulinum toxin type A

1 The axon of the motor nerve innervates the muscular fiber at the motor endplate. Inside the axon terminal, vacuoles of acetyl choline are stored.
2 After electric stimulus of the motor neuron, the acetyl choline vacuoles bind with the SNARE complex that is attached to the presynaptic membrane.
3 Binding of the vacuole to the SNARE complex results in conformational change, directing the vacuole to the membrane.
4 The vacuole fuses with the presynaptic membrane and its contents are released into the synaptic cleft.
5 The neurotransmitter acetyl choline diffuses to the postsynaptic membrane and binds to its target receptor, resulting in contraction of the muscle fiber.

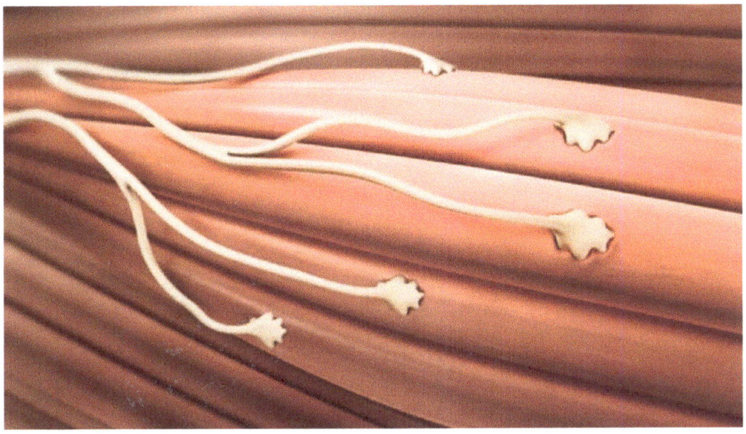

Watch video at http://bit.ly/botulinum-toxin-in-aesthetic-medicine-uma-academy
Movie kindly provided by Merz Aesthetics

Video 1
Mechanism of action of botulinum toxin type A

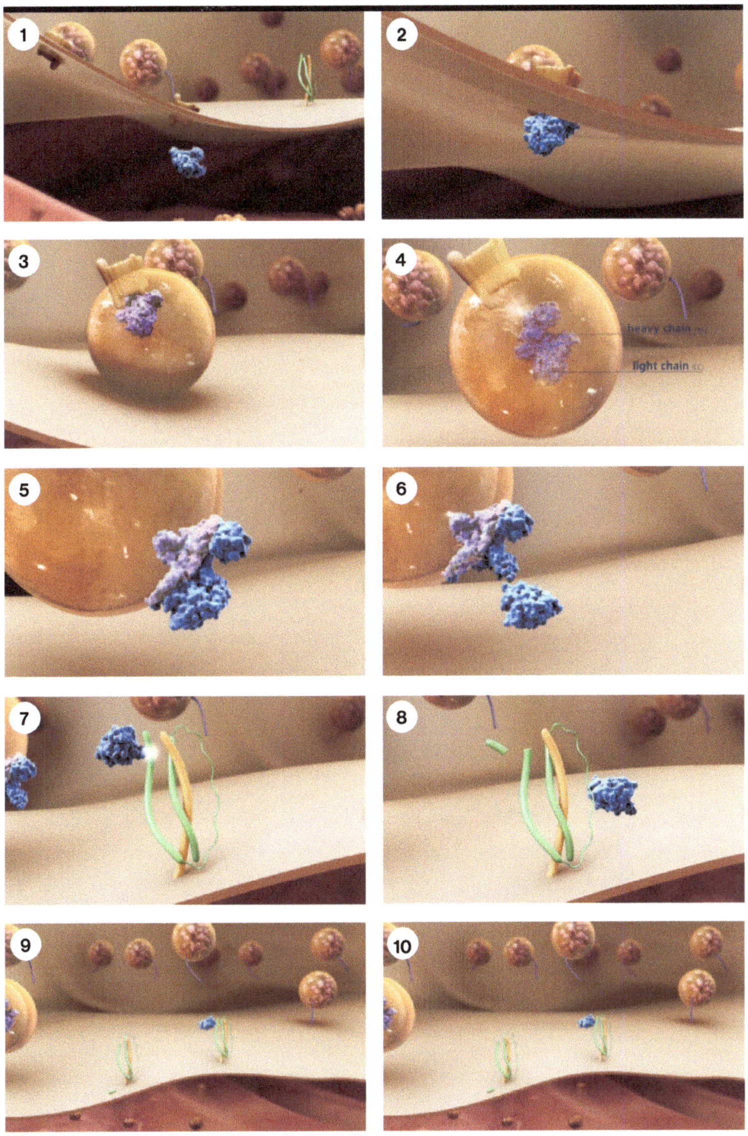

Images kindly provided by Merz Aesthetics

Figure 2
Mechanism of action of botulinum toxin type A

1 The botulinum toxin dipeptide binds to the presynaptic membrane receptor SV2.
2 After binding, endocytosis is initiated.
3 An endocytosis vacuole is released from the plasma membrane and free in the cytosol.
4 The pH lowers and causes the heavy chain to dissociate from the light chain.
5 Due to the low pH, the heavy chain forms a transmembrane protein in the endocytosis vacuole membrane and allows the light chain to pass through its pore.
6 The light chain is released and diffuses freely through the cytosol.
7 The light chain specifically cleaves the SNAP-25 protein, which is part of the SNARE complex.
8 The light chain, being a protease, retains its activity after cleaving.
9 Additional SNAP-25 proteins are cleaved by the same light chain.
10 After electric stimulus of the motor neuron, no binding is possible with the SNARE complex due to the cleaved SNAP-25 protein. No nero-transmitter is released into the synaptic cleft and no muscular contraction is the result.

1.3 Training and continuing medical education

The Dutch Society of Aesthetic Medicine has developed a 2-year post-graduate medical profile specialty training program for physicians who want to specialize in aesthetic medicine. This full-time training program covers injectables, cosmetic dermatology, energy-based devices and (knowledge of) aesthetic surgery. The Dutch authorities have officially approved this training program as it is structured according to the CAN-MEDS system and therefore meets the highest standards of medical specialist training. As many countries do not have official specialist training in aesthetic medicine or aesthetic botulinum toxin therapy, we advise practitioners to follow courses that assess theoretical and technical skills, and to keep a logbook as proof of experience, as legislation concerning who is allowed to perform these treatments is becoming stricter around the globe. Proof of knowledge of cosmetic surgery, fillers, biostimulators, threads, mesotherapy, platelet-rich plasma, needling, cosmeceuticals, dermato-pathology, chemical peels, lasers, intense-pulsed light, focused ultrasound and other energy-based devices is also strongly recommended in order to advise patients on the appropriate therapies and individualized treatment.

Maintaining theoretical knowledge and technical skills is a prerequisite for quality of care. A minimum number of treatments and days per week working with botulinum toxin can assure the quality of the practitioner. On average, the doctor should work at least 2 days per week in aesthetic medicine and treat at least 5 patients per week with botulinum toxin. Theoretical knowledge can be maintained by visiting aesthetic congresses, e-learning and workshops. Certificates of attendance should be kept as proof of the respective society's accreditation.

We advise practitioners to follow courses that assess theoretical and technical skills, and to keep a logbook as proof of experience, as legislation concerning who is allowed to perform these treatments is becoming stricter around the globe.

1.4 Manufacturers

There are three manufacturers who have marketed botulinum toxin type A (botulinum toxin) in Europe. Each of the manufacturers has a product with registration for neurological indications as well as a product for cosmetic indications (Table 1).

The different manufacturers all use the same strain of Clostridium Botulinum (the so-called "Hall strain") and therefore, in principle, produce the same botulinum toxin type A molecule. The pharmacologically active protein should therefore be identical in these products and the same clinical effects should be achieved. However, there are variations in the production process so that the final products are different from each other. The Merz Aesthetics products, Bocouture® and Xeomin®, are free from complexing proteins, containing only the core botulinum neurotoxin type A. The products of Allergan and Ipsen contain botulinum neurotoxin type A and complexing proteins, which have no pharmaco-logical effect. When the these products are reconstituted in saline at physiological pH, the complexing proteins dissociate from the botulinum neurotoxin so that in all products, the free botulinum neurotoxin is present prior to injection.

The determination of units is undertaken by each manu-facturer with their own proprietary LD50 assay. These assays differ and therefore the units are not necessarily equal. Several studies suggest that the conversion factor between Merz and Allergan is 1:1 and between Allergan (or Merz) and Ipsen is 1:2.5. A striking difference is the amount of albumin per vial (see Table 1). It is possible that the relatively low amount of albumin in the Ipsen products Azzalure® and Dysport® is the reason why Ipsen units require a conversion factor.

Table 1
Manufacturers and botulinum toxin products
U: international units sU: Speywood units.

Manufacturer	Brand	Content	Indication
01 **Merz Aesthetics** Scientific name: IncobotulinumtoxinA	Bocouture®	50 U or 100 U per vial	Glabella Periorbital lines Horizontal forehead lines
	Xeomin®	100 U per vial	Neurological
02 **Allergan** Scientific name: OnabotulinumtoxinA	Vistabel®	50 U per vial	Glabella Periorbital lines Horizontal forehead lines
	Botox®	100 U per vial	Neurological
03 **Ipsen** Scientific name: AbobotulinumtoxinA	Azzalure®	125 sU per vial	Glabella Periorbital lines
	Dysport®	500 sU per vial	Neurological

general

Table 2
Product characteristics and differences

	Dysport® / Azzalure®	**Xeomin® / Bocouture®**	**Botox® / Vistabel®**
Active Ingredient	Botulinum neurotoxin type A	Botulinum neurotoxin type A	Botulinum neurotoxin type A
Other clostridial proteins	Hemagglutinin Proteins Flaggelin		Non-toxic, non-hemagglutinin proteins and hemagglutinin proteins
Molecular weight	500-900 kDa	150 kDa	900 kDa
Additional ingredients	Albumin 0.125 mg Lactose 2.5 mg	Albumin 1 mg Sucrose 4.7 mg	Albumin 0.5 mg NaCl 0.5 mg
Total proteins	ca. 4.35 ng/500 sU	ca. 0.44 ng/100 U	ca. 5 ng/100 U
Units conversion factor	1:2.5	1	1
Mechanism of action	SNAP-25	SNAP-25	SNAP-25
Official indications	Glabella, Lateral Periorbital lines	Glabella, Lateral Periorbital lines, Horizontal forehead lines	Glabella, Lateral Periorbital lines, Forehead lines
Product Form	Powder	Powder (freeze-dried)	Powder
Dosage per vial	125 Speywood U/vial	50 Merz U/vial 100 Merz U/vial	50 Allergan U/vial
Reconstitution	0.9% NaCl	0.9% NaCl	0.9% NaCl
Recommended number of units per 0.1 ml	20	4	4
Storage temperature unopened vial	Cooled: 2-8°C	Lower than 25°C	Cooled: 2-8°C
Shelf life unopened flacon	Not mentioned	36 months	36 months
Storage temperature after reconstitution	Cooled: 2-8°C	Cooled: 2-8°C	Cooled: 2-8°C
Shelf life after reconstitution	4 hours	24 hours	24 hours

1.5 Diffusion and spread of botulinum toxin products

Diffusion of botulinum toxin is about moving the molecules from the injection site, on the basis of the concentration difference of the botulinum toxin with respect to the surrounding tissue. The speed of diffusion of botulinum toxin is dependent on molecule size, and will stop after binding to its target receptor (SV2).

Several publications have shown differences in diffusion radii of botulinum toxin products; in particular, differences between the products of Ipsen and Allergan have been widely described. Ipsen appears to have a larger diffusion radius than the Allergan botulinum toxin. Allergan and Merz products have a similar diffusion profile. Due to the fact that, after reconstitution, the complexing proteins dissociate from the toxin within one minute, the expla-nations for differences in diffusion are not related to the molecular size of the protein complex; the 900 kDa molecule of Allergan has an identical diffusion profile to the 150 kDa molecule of Merz.

Spread of botulinum toxin is a clinical observation that differs from diffusion. Physical forces such as massage, injection techniques, dilution volumes, thickness and length of the injection needle, etc. influence spread. In one study, the three products were compared on the basis of their anhidrotic halo with the Azzalure®/ Dysport® product appearing to have a larger spread than the other two products. Other studies indicate an equal distribution.

1.6 Reconstitution of botulinum toxin products

According to the instructions for use, the three different products must be reconstituted in physiologic saline solution (0.9% NaCl) to 0.1 ml per 4U (Merz and Allergan) or 20 sU (Ipsen). The medical literature has published various methods to make the injections less painful, such as adding lidocaine and using bacteriostatic saline (in which benzyl alcohol is added for an anesthetic effect).

1 **Reconstitution of Azzalure®**
   0.63 ml saline (whether or not buffered) per vial of 125 sU in order to obtain a concentration of 5sU / 0.05 ml.

2 **Reconstitution of Vistabel®**
   1.25 ml saline per vial of 50 U in order to obtain a concentration of 4U / 0.1 ml.

3 **Reconstitution of Bocouture®**
   1.25 ml NaCl (whether or not buffered) per vial of 50U or 2.5 ml in a vial of 100U in order to obtain a concentration of 4U / 0.1 ml. For Bocouture® it is recommended to gently pivot the vial, and to make sure that the saline has touched all the surfaces on the inside of the vial, including the rubber cap. Due to the manufacturing proccess, the botulinum toxin can be anywhere in the vials, incluing the afore mentioned surfaces. If, after reconstitution, the solution is cloudy or contains visible particles, the solution should not be used.

Diffusion of botulinum toxin is about moving the molecules from the injection site, on the basis of the concentration difference of the botulinum toxin with respect to the surrounding tissue.

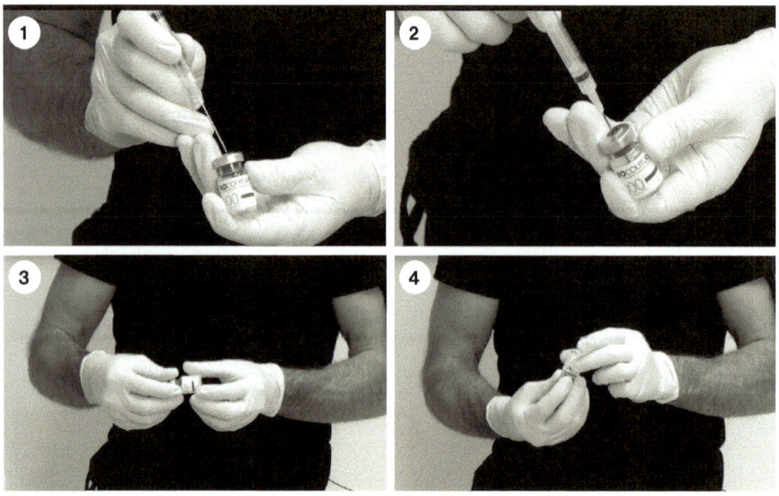

Figure 3
Reconstitution of Bocouture®

1. Fill a syringe with 2.5 mL of (bacteriostatic) saline and attach a 18G needle.
2. When the needle is advanced through the rubber cap, the vacuum inside the vial pulls the cotents of the syringe into the vial.
3. After removing the needle, swirl the saline by rolling the vial.
4. Make sure the saline touches everywhere inside the vial, including the rubber cap to assure all neurotoxin gets into the solution.

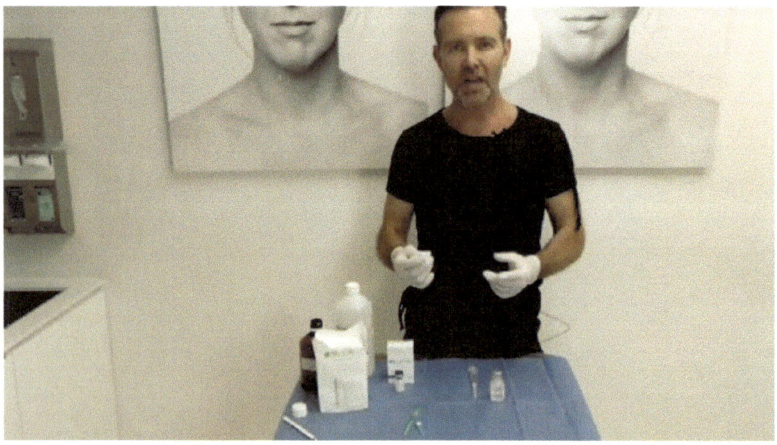

Video 2
Reconstitution of Bocouture®

Watch video at http://bit.ly/botulinum-toxin-in-aesthetic-medicine-uma-academy

1.7 Contra indications

Absolute contra indications

1. Fever or feeling sick
2. Permanent filler in the treatment area
3. Hypersensitivity to botulinum toxin type A or any product used as a component
4. Myasthenia Gravis, Eaton Lambert Syndrome or other muscle activity disorders in medical history
5. Pregnancy or lactation
6. Infection in the treatment area
7. Melanoma or other malignancy in the treatment area

Relative contra indications

1. Skin diseases or inflammation in treatment area
2. Coagulation disorders
3. The use of anti-coagulation, in association with an increased risk of bruises
4. The presence of ALS or peripheral neuromuscular disorders
5. Body Dysmorphic Disorder
6. Specific additional treatments in the treatment area, before or after the botulinum toxin treatment
7. Aminoglycoside antibiotics or drugs affecting neuromuscular transmission (for example tubocurarine-type muscle relaxants)
8. Permanent fillers around the treatment area

1.8 Patient consultation and documentation

A good understanding of the wishes of the patient is essential. The physician should create and verify realistic expectations of the possible results and complication risks. During consultation, a mirror or photographs can be used to specify the treatment areas and expected results, limitations of the botulinum toxin treatment, and pointing out pre-existing asymmetries. The types of wrinkles (dynamic, static), their etiologies and treatment options should be explained. All relevant information should be entered in the patient file. A thourough patient history must also be documented in the patient file and should include information on general health, pregnancy, lactation, allergies, use of medication and contra indications.

There are cultural differences between different patient subgroups affecting beauty ideals. European patients generally want a subtle, natural and fresh look, not necessarily a frozen or mask face appearance. The underlying reason for this is that this will improve self-confidence and overall quality of life. The treatment dose is at the discretion of the practitioner on the basis of individual anatomy and to the wishes of the patient. The abovementioned key messages should be communicated to patients and it should be documented that the patient has received this information.

1.9 Patient information

- **Mechanism of action:** Botulinum toxin causes weakening of the treated muscle. The muscle recovers fully from this temporary weakening after several months. Botulinum toxin is a protein that temporarily blocks the signal transmission between nerve and muscle.
- **Duration of effect:** The relaxation of the treated muscles starts to become noticeable after a few days and is at its maximum after about 2-4 weeks. The effect lasts about 3-4 months (by repeating the treatment, the effect may last longer when the muscle is not fully recovered from the previous treatment and the effect may last shorter if the dose is reduced).
- **Treatment repetition:** Treatment should be repeated after about 3-4 months, but not earlier due to the potential for immunogenicity to botulinum toxin in the case of Vistabel or Azzalure. Bocouture®/Xeomin® does not have an increased risk of immunogenicity and so the 3 months interval limitation is not mentioned in the instructions for use.

1.10 Complications and side effects

01

Headaches
Some patients may have headaches and flu-like symptoms for several days. These side effects are very rare.

02

Local side effects
Local side effects can be expected such as injection pain, redness, bruising and possibly a small amount of bleeding at the injection site.

03

Unintended muscle effect
An adjacent muscle can be affected unintentionally, thus an unintended aesthetic effect may occur (frontalis muscle: brow ptosis; m. levator palpebrae: levatorptosis (dropped eyelid); zygomaticus major muscle: altered smile). If there is insufficient effect, a touch-up treatment can be performed after 2 weeks.

04

Allergic reaction
Allergic reactions are very rare (less than 0.1%).

general

1.11 Pre and post procedure

Informed consent

A treatment agreement must meet the following characteristics:

1. Patient expressly consents to treatment and acknowledges assumption of risks.
2. It must be in writing (digital or print).
3. It has to contain the date and the signature of the patient.
4. It must be signed before the treatment.
5. Some countries adhere to a cooling-off period of 24 hours.

Photography

Photography represents an integral part of the aesthetic patient file. A patient must consent to having their image taken before being photographed. Take photos in relaxed and dynamic states, from different angles, and in a standardized manner.

Facial analysis and physical examination

During the physical examination the position of the eyebrows, the degree of dynamic wrinkles, the appearance of the skin, volume (loss), creases, folds, scars, etc. should be analyzed and discussed with the patient. Attention should be paid to potential malignant lesions (eg melanoma) and other skin pathologies that are contra indications for injection. Analysis of facial muscles should be performed in relaxed and dynamic states: while frowning, raising eyebrows and squinting. During facial analysis, pay attention to symmetry, anatomical features of the muscles and the pattern of lines and wrinkles. Based on muscular anatomy, marking of the injection points is performed immediately prior to injection with the patient positioned on the treatment chair.

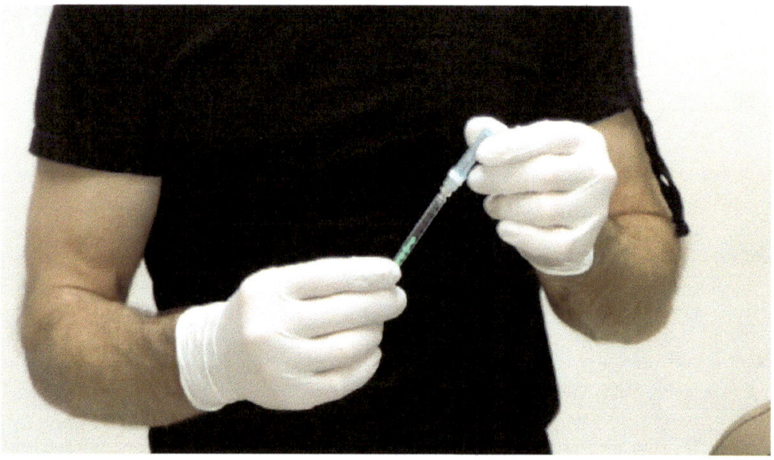

Video 3
Facial assessment and anatomical background prior to botulinum toxin treatment

Watch video at http://bit.ly/botulinum-toxin-in-aesthetic-medicine-uma-academy

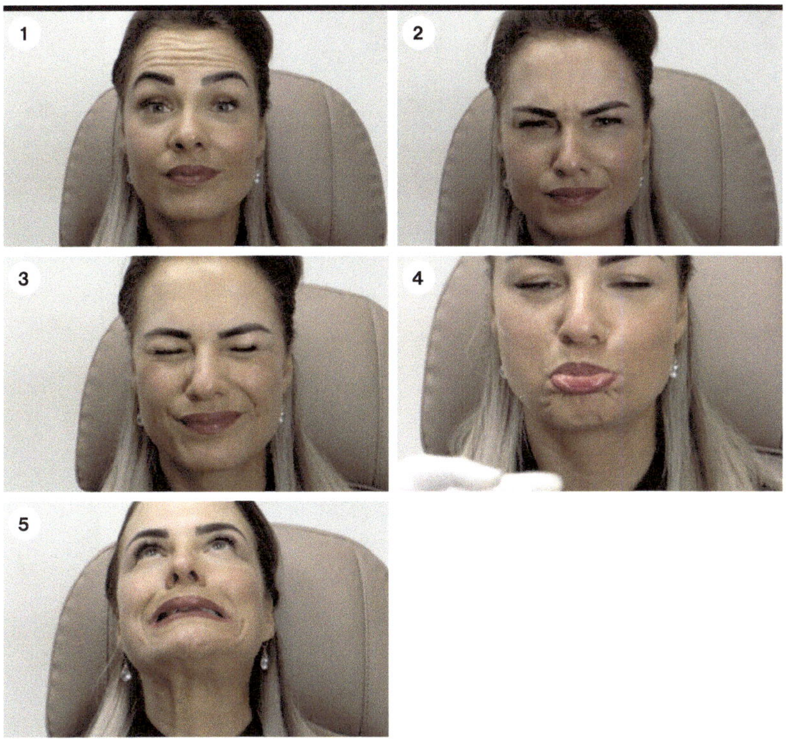

Figure 4
Facial assessment

1 Assessment of the frontalis muscle.
2 Assessment of the glabella.
3 Assessment of the orbicularis oculi muscle.
4 Assessment of the mentalis muscle.
5 Assessment of the depressor anguli oris muscle and the platysma.

Patient preparation

If required, topical creams, vibration devices or cooling can be considered for anesthesia. Position the patient in a comfortable treatment chair with proper lighting. General infection prevention measures should be used including wearing disposable gloves and disinfecting the skin prior to injection.

After care

Many experts advise their patients to properly frown and flex the treated muscles for 1 hour after treatment in order for the toxin to bind at the target receptor. However, no evidence was found to support this statement. In fact, the basic tonus of the muscle may be sufficient to allow for binding of the protein to its receptor. Patients are advised not to rub their eyes, not to touch, rub or press the injection site, have facial massages, do strenuous exercise, bend or lay down, sunbathe, visit a sauna, or consume alcohol for several hours after the treatment, in order to minimize spread. This well-meant advice is not evidence-based, but no harm is done when advising patients of this after care.

1.12 General injection techniques

The following injection techniques are generally used for botulinum toxin treatment:

01

Intramuscular bolus technique

With this widely-used technique the point of the needle is placed directly through the skin into the muscle at a location where a high concentration of motor endplates is presumed to be present. The needle tip is not displaced while the botulinum toxin is injected.

02

Subcutaneous bolus injection technique

This technique is used when the risk of passing through a superficial muscle needs to be minimized, for example in the platysma muscle

03

Intradermal bolus injection technique

This technique is used when the risk for an underlying blood vessel or diffusion radius needs to be minimized, for example in the forehead.

04

Retrograde injection technique

This technique is used when spread must be controlled, for example in the mentalis muscle, the orbicularis oris muscle, or the orbicularis oculi muscle.

05

Microtoxin injection technique

This technique is often used with hyperdiluted botulinum toxin; when the dose has to be very low and superficial, for example in the risorius muscle, forehead and lateral cheeks.

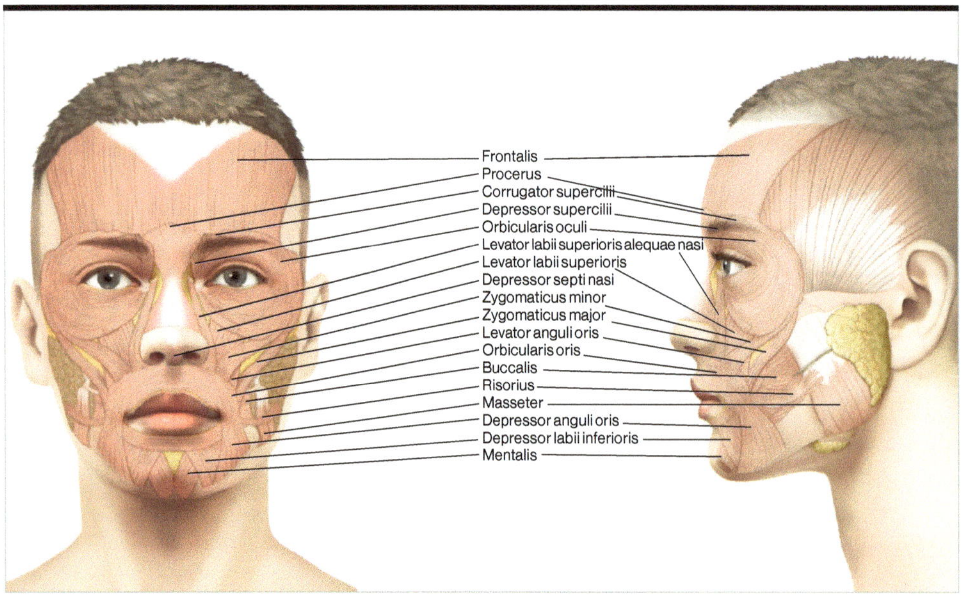

Figure 5
Facial muscles

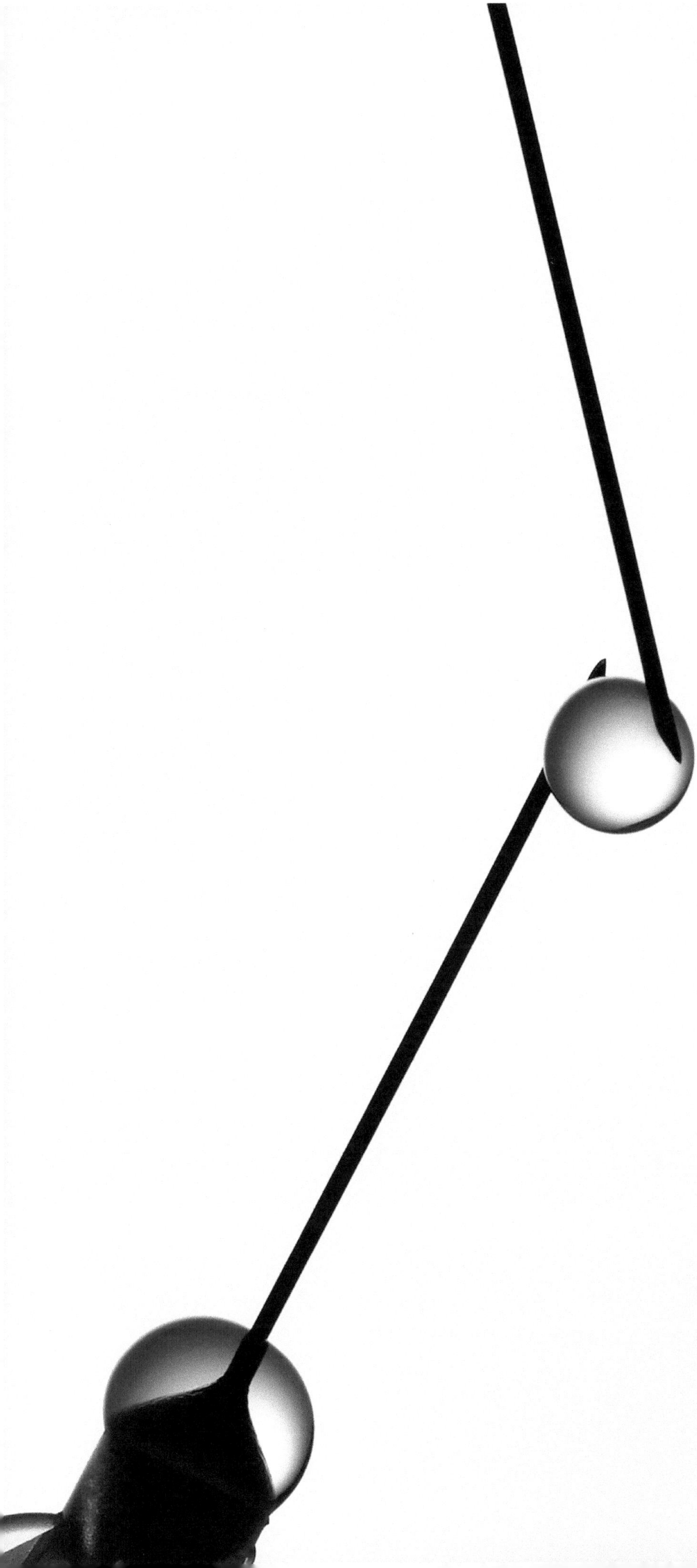

02
upper third of the face

introduction

Muscles of facial expression maintain a balance of the mimetic movements in the face. In the upper third of the face, there are two types of muscles: levators and depressors. The frontalis muscle is the only levator for the eyebrows, while the procerus, corrugator supercillii, depressor supercillii and the orbicularis oculi muscles are the depressors. This chapter describes the treatment protocols for each of the abovementioned muscles, respecting the balance of the eyebrows.

upper third of the face

2.1 Horizontal forehead lines (frontalis muscle)

The injection pattern of the frontalis muscle is shown in figure below. Generally, 4 to 6 injections are administered with 2 U / 5 sU per injection site at a depth of approximately 2-3 mm using an intramuscular, subcutaneous or intradermal injection technique. The first injection site can be marked at 3-4 cm cranial to the orbital rim, from the peak of the brow along the direction of the muscle fibers. The second point is found vertically from the medial canthus, at about 3-4 cm above the orbital rim. The third injection site is found between the first two points, also 3-4 cm above the orbital rim. Besides these three injection points per side, micro intradermal injections can be performed with approximately 0.5 U / 1.25 sU per microinjection to prevent any residual horizontal wrinkles.

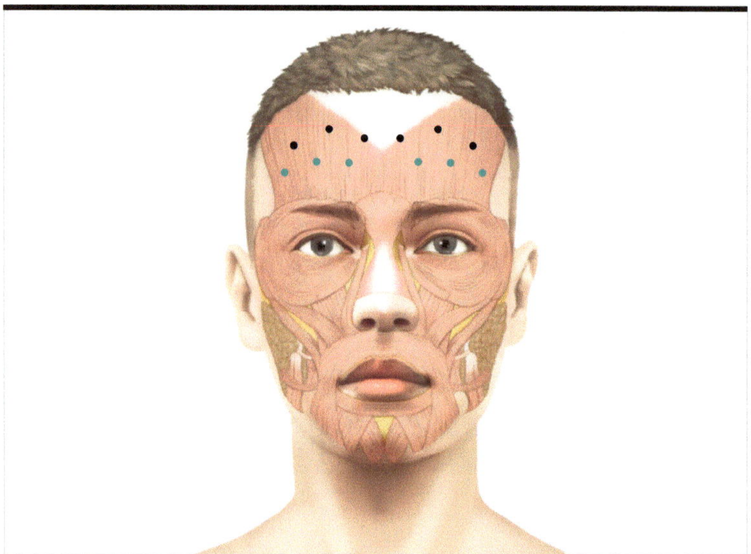

Figure 6
Injections horizontal forehead lines (frontalis muscle)

Black: the most common sites of injection (subcutaneous bolus injection technique) of about 2 U / 5 sU per injection site;
Blue: additional possible injection sites (intradermal injection technique) of about 0.5-1 U / 1.25 sU per injection site.

As the frontalis muscle is the only levator muscle of the eyebrows, a relative overdose can result in a brow ptosis. To prevent brow ptosis, injections in the lower half of the frontalis muscle should be avoided.

Dosage frontal dynamic wrinkles

The dosage for men is different from the dosage for women with men generally receiving a higher dosage due to larger muscle development.

	Dose	Number of injection sites
Men	6-20 U / 20-60 sU	4-12
Women	6-16 U / 20-60 sU	4-12

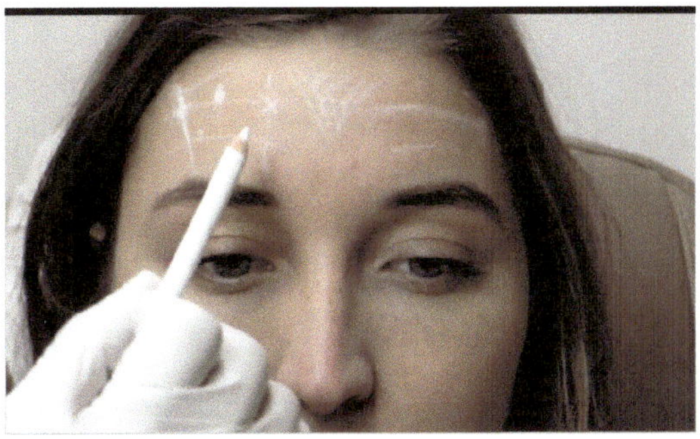

Figure 7
Horizontal forehead lines

Intramascular as well as intradermal botulinum toxin injections

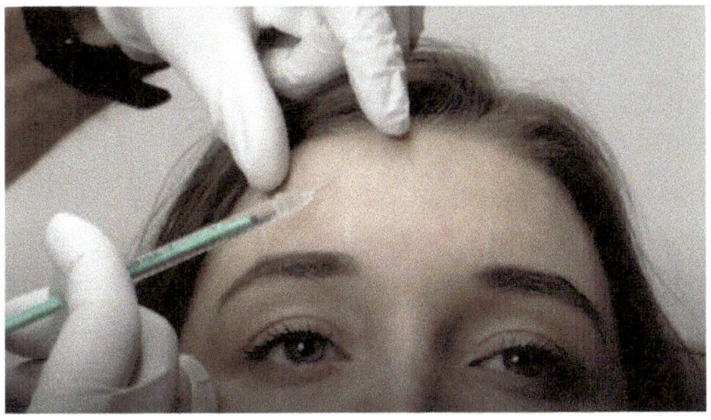

Video 4
Horizontal forehead lines standard protocol

Watch video at http://bit.ly/botulinum-toxin-in-aesthetic-medicine-uma-academy

2.2 Personal tweaks with Bocouture® / Xeomin®

Having adapted the new insights of fibroblast contraction, we hyperdilute Xeomin® to approximately 6 ml saline / 100 U. When using 10 U for the forehead, (0.25 ml), we add 0.35 ml, to get a volume of 0.6 ml per 10 U. This gives most significant fibroblast contraction and may result in increased lift. The injections are performed intradermally and also have an effect on the frontalis muscle. The dose and injection points remain the same, or more points can be added to assure a homogeneous distribution of the product. If needed, the dose can be increased in the upper forehead at follow-up visits to further reduce muscle strength.

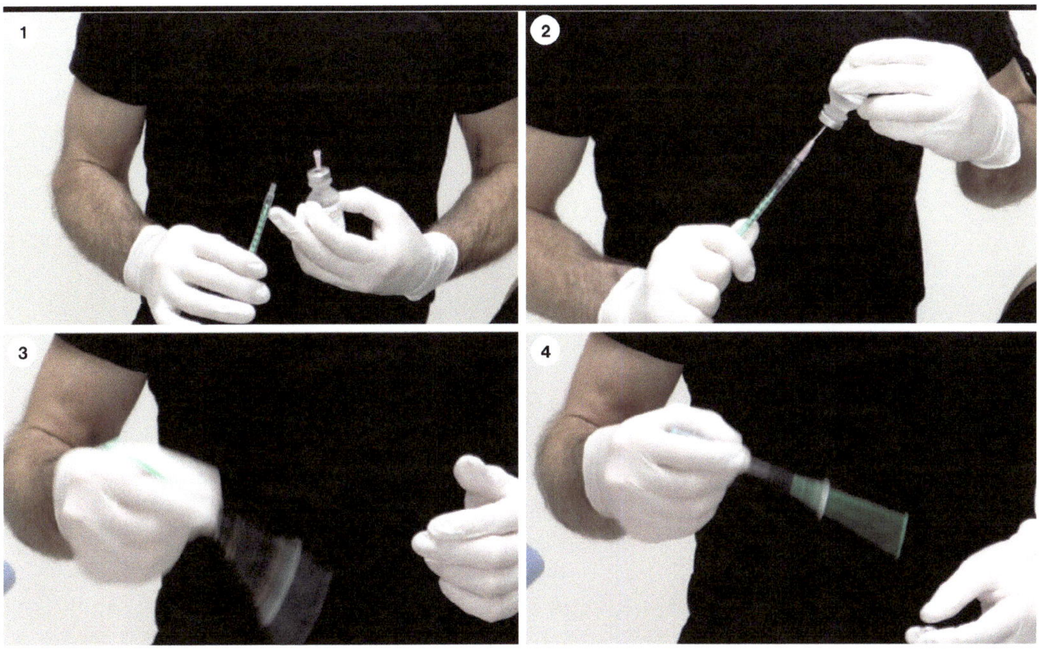

Figure 8
Hyperdiluting Bocouture®/Xeomin®

1. In this case, 12 U for the forehead was chosen.
2. The ideal dose is 6 ml / 100 U = 0,72 ml / 12 U, so add saline until approximately 0,7 ml.
3. Leaving an air bubble in the syringe, gently centrifuge the bubble to the other side.
4. Repeat a few times for homogeneous solution.

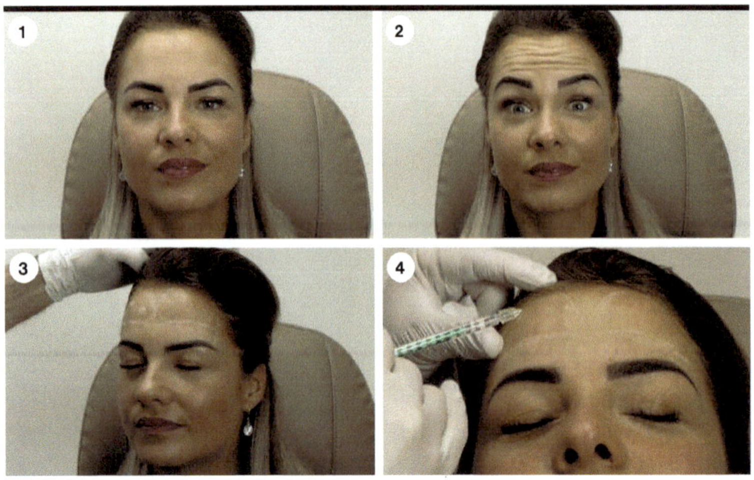

Figure 9
Intradermal injection of hyperdiluted botulinum toxin

1. Frontalis muscle in relaxed states.
2. Frontalis muscle in contracted states.
3. Marking each marked point, in this case hyper diluted Bocouture® (100 U / 6 ml).
4. Injecting each marked point, in this case hyper diluted Bocouture® (100 U / 6 ml).

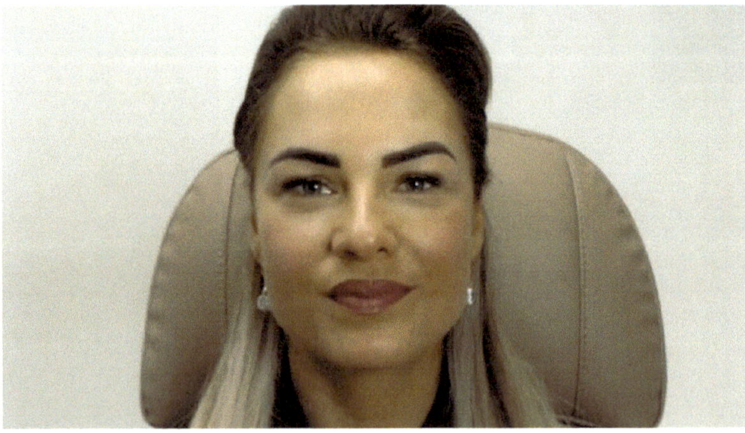

Video 5
Intradermal injection of hyperdiluted botulinum toxin

Watch video at http://bit.ly/botulinum-toxin-in-aesthetic-medicine-uma-academy

2.3 GRID21 and Grid ONE21 methods

A relatively new bespoke treatment option is using the GRID21 method. This is an individualized treatment approach for the frontalis muscle designed by Dr. Phillip Levy where the muscles are injected in up to 21 points with varying dosages in every point depending on muscular strength at those points and the desired eyebrow shape. An alternative, but similar, approach of the GRID21 method, is the ONE21 technique, developed by Dr. Carla de Sanctis Pecora et. al. It is a safe technique for the treatment of forehead wrinkles with a predictable eyebrow reshape. This protocol considers both clinical as well as anatomical patterns shown by the patient. Pre-treatment assessment of the upper face, grading of wrinkles, muscle strength, and patient request for eyebrow shape and positioning will determine the dosage for each injection points.

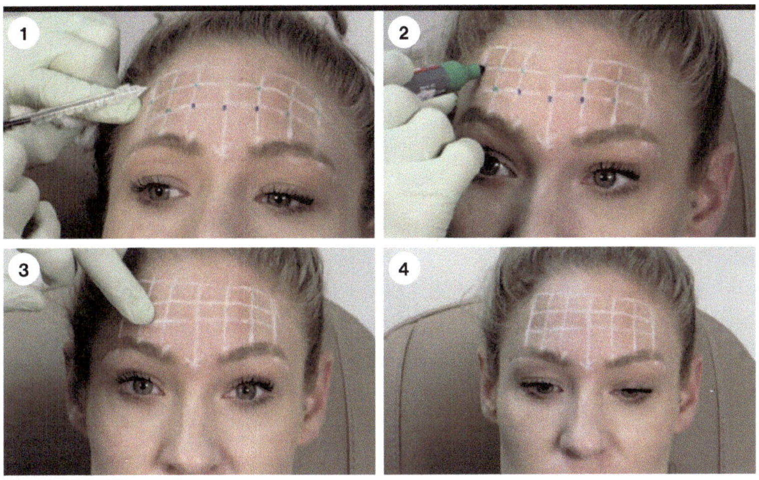

Figure 10
GRID21 method and ONE21 technique

Each point is marked with a specific dose depending on the individual muscular strength in 21 points on the forehead.

1. Marking of the grid: midline, medial canthus, mid-pupillary line, lateral canthus (vertical) and the lowest wrinkle ("Inferior Limit Line"), the highest wrinkle and a line in between (horizontal).
2. Feeling per individual intersection point the strength of the muscle.
3. By applying low, intermediate and high pressure on each individual grid point with the finger tips, the corresponding effect on the brow position can be assessed. Then, marking with corresponding colors for low, intermediate or high dose can be done per injection point.
4. Performing the injections. In this example, red = 2 U, blue = 1 U and green = 0.5 U.

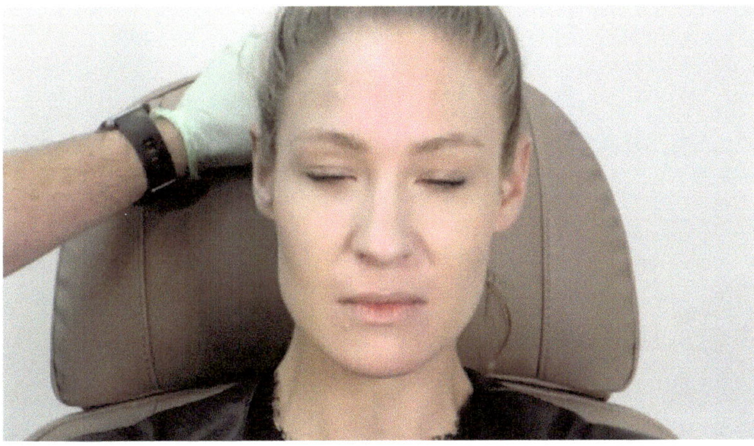

Video 6
GRID21 method and ONE21 technique

Watch video at http://bit.ly/botulinum-toxin-in-aesthetic-medicine-uma-academy

upper third of the face

Complications

01

Brow ptosis

As the frontalis muscle is the only levator muscle of the eyebrows, a relative overdose can result in a lower position of the brows. The recommendation is therefore to inject the depressors of the brow in the same treatment session: procerus, depressor supercilii, orbicularis oculi and corrugator supercilii muscles. To prevent brow ptosis, injections in the lower half of the frontalis muscle should be avoided. Superficial injection is also advisable. When botulinum toxin enters into the subgaleal glide space it may easily spread caudally. Inside the muscle there are many blood vessels. If the needle punctures the vessel wall and blood flows into the surrounding tissue, more spread can be expected. Treatment of brow ptosis consists of weakening the depressors (see 'brow lift').

02

Hematoma / ecchymosis

The temporal, supraorbital and supratrochlear arteries and their branches run through the treatment area, as well as small and large veins. Good inspection is therefore important to prevent hematomas. Injecting intradermally reduces the risk of puncturing blood vessels.

03

Mephisto look

The Mephisto look, also known as the Jack Nicholson eyebrow, is characterized by medial depression and lateral elevation of the eyebrow. The cause is a reactive hyper-contraction of the lateral part of the frontalis muscle by relaxation of the medial part of the frontalis muscle. Treatment consists of the injection of 1-2 U / 2.5-5 sU in the fibers of the lateral frontalis muscle.

2.4 Glabella (various muscles)

The muscles that have an effect on the glabellar frown lines are the procerus, the depressor supercilii, the corrugator supercilii and the orbicularis oculi. Procerus: 4-6 U / 10-15 sU is injected in the midline at the level of the superciliary line, where the needle is placed perpendicular to the skin, approximately 6 mm deep (a half-needle). The two depressor supercilii muscles are both treated due to the diffusion radius of about 1 cm at this dosage.
The medial injection of the corrugator supercilii muscle, about 0.5 cm above the base of the eyebrow (at the level of the medial canthus), is given deep at about 8 mm (3/4 needle) due to the medially located origin at the periosteum 4-6 U / 10-15 sU. The lateral injection site is superficial 2-4 mm deep (1/4 needle), directly medial to the skin insertion. The insertion of the corrugator can be found by asking the patient to frown. A depression in the skin (corrugator dimple) marks the place where the muscle fibers pull the skin towards the medial origin. The corrugator is injected 0.5-1 cm outside the orbital rim to avoid brow ptosis and eyelid ptosis.

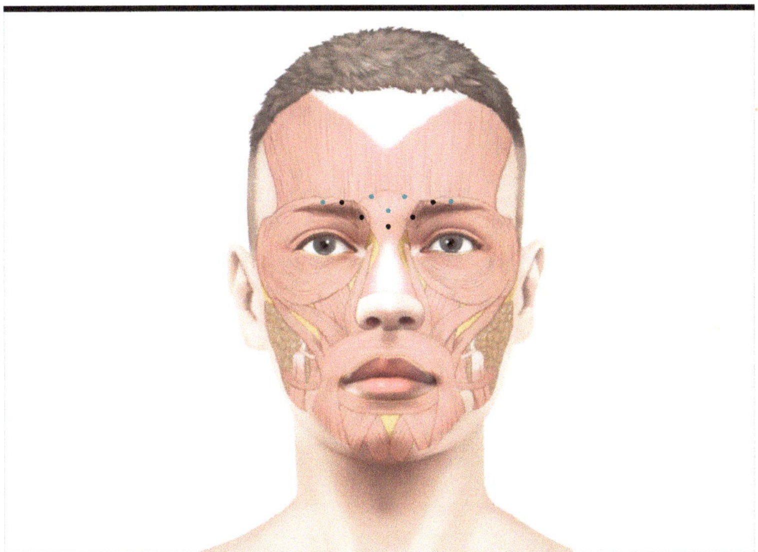

Figure 11
Injections pattern of the glabella

Black: the most common sites of injection (intramuscular injection technique);
Blue: additional possible injection sites (lateral: intradermal technique, be careful of brow ptosis; medial: intramuscular technique).

Dosage Glabella

The dosage for men differs from the dosage for women with men generally receiving a higher dose due to larger muscle development. With men, the corrugator supercilii muscle often runs more laterally.

	Dose	Number of injection sites
Men	24 U / 60 sU	5-7
Women	24 U / 50 sU	5-7

High dose glabella treatment

Building up to the introduction of a new botulinum toxin product on the US market, A recent study showed a positive dose-response relationship with increasing doses of IncobotulinumtoxinA (INCO, Xeomin/Bocouture) for the glabellar frown lines (GFL). This study demonstrated a median duration of effect of 185 days with a dose of 50U INCO and 210 days with 75U INCO. The primary efficacy endpoint was duration of effect was defined as at least one point improvement compared to baseline using the Facial Wrinkle Scale.[61]

It is hypothesized, based on preclinical data, that a higher dose results in a longer duration of effect because more botulinum toxin can bind to the motor endplates, and, with that, more light chain molecules to reach the cytosol of the neuron.[62] Consequently, the degradation will take longer.[63]

Other commercially available botulinum toxin, such as OnabotulinumtoxinA and AbobotulinumtoxinA, have showed similar positive dose-response curves for the treatment of GFL.

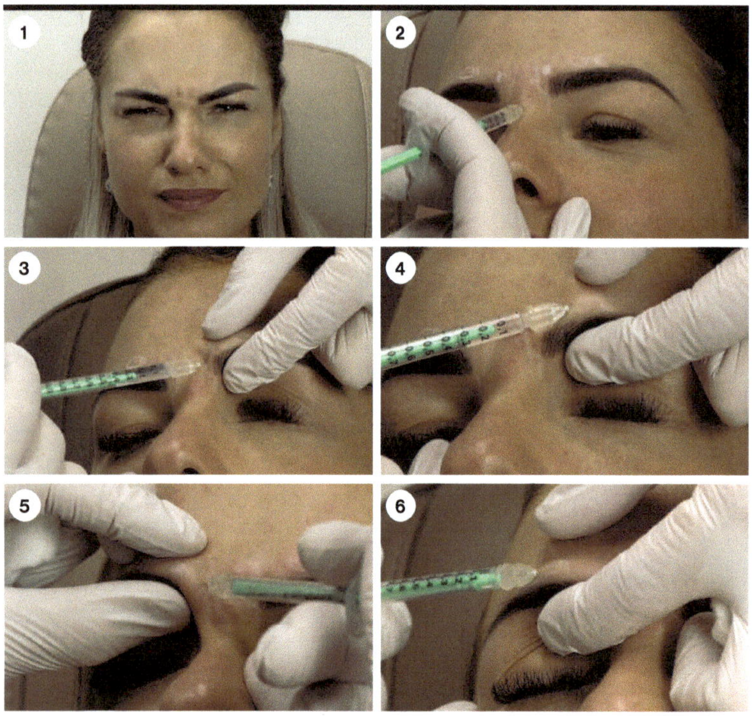

Figure 12
Glabella injections

1	Glabellar complex in contracted state.
2	Markings and procerus muscle injection.
3 and **5**	Deep injection in the medial side of the corrugator supercilii muscle.
4 and **6**	Superficial injection in the lateral side of the corrugator.

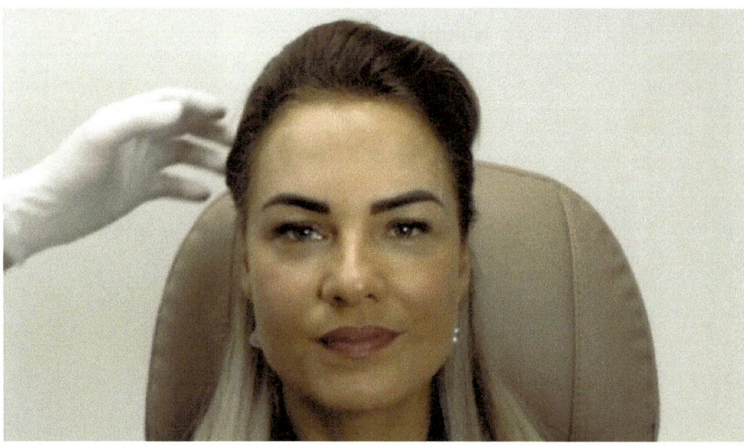

Video 7
Glabella injections

Watch video at http://bit.ly/botulinum-toxin-in-aesthetic-medicine-uma-academy

Complications

01

Mephisto look

The mephisto look is characterized by medial depression and lateral elevation of the eyebrow. The cause is a reactive hyper-contraction of the lateral part of the frontalis muscle by relaxation of the medial part of the frontalis muscle. This is caused by injecting too cranial to the corrugator supercilii muscle resulting in the frontalis muscle being treated as well. It can be avoided by injecting deep into the medial head with a superficial injection in the lateral part of the corrugator supercilii muscle. Corrective treatment requires injection of 1-2 U / 2.5-5 sU in the fibers of the lateral frontalis muscle.

02

Blepharoptosis or levatorptosis

When botulinum toxin enters the intra-orbital space it can reach and weaken the levator palpebrae muscle, causing levator ptosis. The cause of levator ptosis is anatomical in nature; the orbicularis retaining ligament is impermeable to fluid and thereby prevents diffusion or spread to the intra-orbit. However, at the location of the supraorbital notch/foramen an opening exists in this ligament, through which the botulinum toxin can pass. Prevention therefore consists of respecting the distance (0.5-1 cm) from the orbital rim and, in particular, the avoidance of a deep injection near the supraorbital foramen. Treatment includes prescribing eye drops 0.5% apraclonidine three times daily in the affected eye for a maximum of 1 month. Apraclonidine is an agent that is normally intended to reduce the intraocular pressure in case of glaucoma. A side effect of this drug is the effect desired by ptosis: the Müller muscles contract which raise the eyelid 1-3 mm.

03

Brow ptosis

When the lower part of the frontalis muscle is unintentionally weakened, the eyebrow may drop. When injecting the lateral part of the corrugator, the best option is to inject from lateral to medial. In order to prevent brow ptosis, the most lateral border of the corrugator supercilii muscle should be the midpupillary line. Should this complication occur, the depressor muscles can be treated: the orbicularis oculi and lateral corrugator supercilii muscles.

04

Hematoma

The supraorbital and supratrochlear arteries and their branches run through the treatment area, as well as small and large veins. Good inspection is therefore important to prevent hematomas. Intradermal injection reduces the risk of puncturing blood vessels.

2.5 Periorbital wrinkles (orbicularis oculi muscle)

The orbicularis oculi is treated with 3-4 injections of 2-4 U / 5-10 U per injection site. The injection depth is superficial, approximately 2-3 mm (¼ needle) deep, and the pattern is radial, about 1 cm from the orbital rim. Due to the proximity of the bilateral venous plexus, there is a risk of hematomas and the skin needs to be inspected for the course of superficial veins. Cranially, the area of the medial temporal crest should be avoided to prevent influencing the frontalis muscle, and caudally, deep injections should be avoided to prevent influencing the zygomaticus major muscle. Additional intradermal microinjections can be given to treat the finer infraorbital lines.

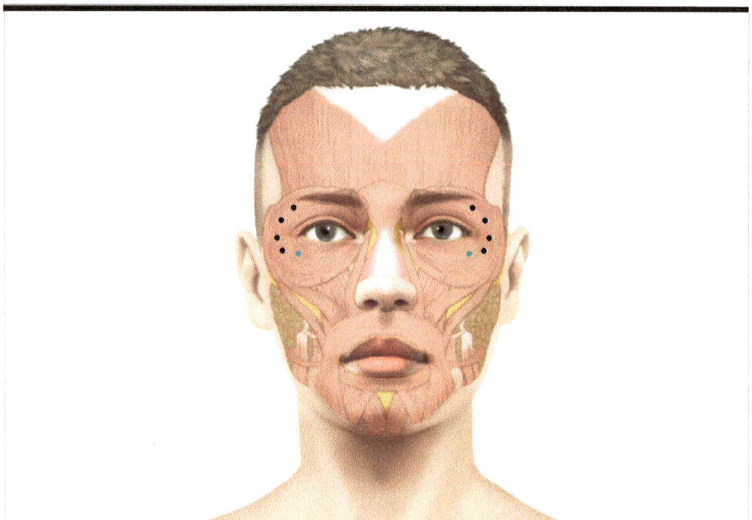

Figure 13
Injection pattern for dynamic periorbital wrinkles

Black: the most common sites of injection (intramuscular injection technique);
Blue: additional possible injection sites (intradermal technique).

Dosage orbicularis oculi muscle
The dosage for men is generally higher than for women due to larger muscle development.

	Average dose	Number of injection sites
Men	20-30 U / 20-60 sU	3-6 per eye
Women	10-30 U / 20-60 sU	3-6 per eye

Complications

01 Brow ptosis

When botulinum toxin is injected too cranially, the caudal area of the frontalis muscle can be affected. As a result, this eyebrow levator muscle will relax and the lateral eyebrow may be lowered. This complication can be avoided by choosing a lateral injection site closer to the brow. Should it occur, the complication can be treated by injecting the orbicularis oculi muscle at the temporal crest.

02 Diplopia

When the needle is inserted through the orbicularis retaining ligament, botulinum toxin can diffuse to the intraorbital muscles that control eye movements causing diplopia. To prevent this complication, it is recommended to keep a minimum distance of 1 cm from the orbital rim.

03 Drooping mouth

If botulinum toxin affects the zygomaticus major muscle (or in extremely rare cases the zygomaticus minor muscle), this will affect the position of the oral commissure. The zygomaticus major muscle has its origin in the periosteum of the zygomatic bone and therefore deep to the orbicularis oculi muscle. Prevention is by avoiding deep injections in this area. Treatment consists of relaxing the antagonist, which is the depressor anguli oris muscle.

04 Hematoma

The venous plexuses in the orbital area pose a significant risk for hematoma. Proper inspection of the skin with a good examination lamp is essential. Treatment consists of direct compression.

05 Eye bags

When the lower eyelids are treated, the tonus of the orbicularis oculi muscle might be weakened in such a way that it bulges anteriorly due to pressure of the underlying fat. To prevent this complication, the dose of toxin for the lower eyelids should be limited to a maximum of 1 U / 2.5 sU per injection site.

Infraorbital bags may also occur as a result of lymphatic stasis causing edema. The orbicularis oculi muscle has a pumping function for the drainage of lymphatic fluid. When this pump is weakened by toxin, stasis and accumulation of lymphatic fluid may result. To prevent this occurring minimal dosage should be used. This side effect is self-limiting and usually disappears within 2 weeks as the lymphatic system will adjust to the new circumstances. Manual lymphatic drainage can also help disperse the fluid.

upper third of the face

2.6 Brow Lift (various muscles)

The brow depressors are all treated at the level of the eyebrow. In addition to the standard glabella injection sites, treatment includes two lateral injections in the orbicularis oculi muscle of about 2-4 U / 5-10 sU each. The lateral injections should not be administered above the level of the eyebrow to avoid influencing the frontalis muscle.

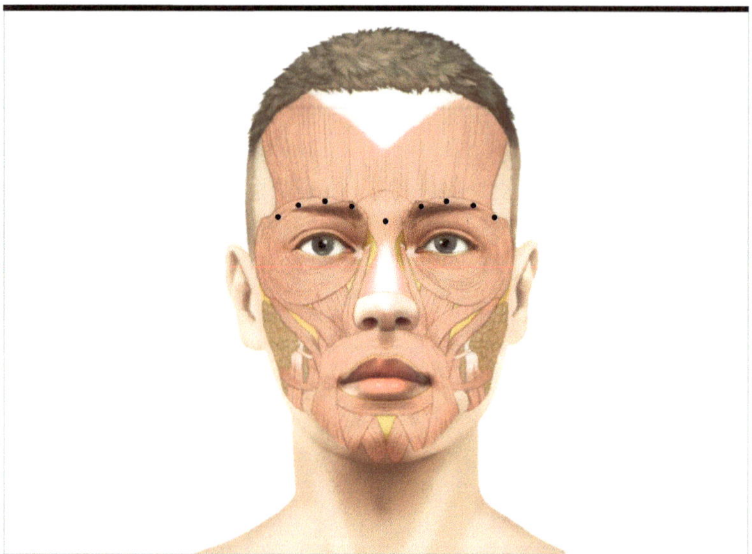

Figure 14
Injection pattern for brow lift

Toxin is administered at 2-4 U / 5-10 sU per injection site (intramuscular injection technique) and injected directly into or caudal to the eyebrow laterally and into or just cranial to the eyebrow medially in combination with procerus injection.

2.7 Tension headache and migraine

Targeting the glabella, frontalis and/or orbicularis oculi muscles in combination with the temporalis muscle is often effective for the treatment of tension headache. The temporalis muscle can be treated by four injections and a total of 16-32 U / 40-80 sU per side, with the injection points about 2-3 cm apart. Injections should be deep as the temporalis muscle lies just above the periosteum, underneath the deep temporal fascia (temporalis muscle aponeurosis). Palpate before treatment to locate the superficial temporal artery. In some individuals the masseter muscle may also contribute to headaches. Injection of this muscle is described in the section on masseter hypertrophy. Finally, in some patients, the trapezius and occipitalis muscles may contribute to tension headaches and migraines. However, treatment of these muscles is beyond the scope of these protocols. The temporalis muscle is often hypertrophic in patients with tension headaches and migraines. Therefore, treatment of this primarily medical condition has an aesthetic goal as well and is therefore included in this book.

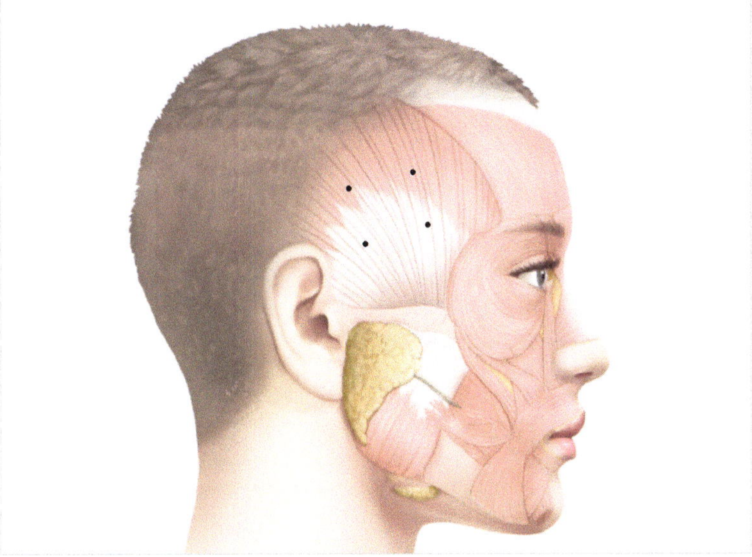

Figure 15
Injection technique for the temporalis muscle for treatment of migraine

Inject the temporalis muscle with an intramuscular bolus technique using 4-8 U / 10-20 sU per injectio and spacing injection points approximately 2-3 cm apart.

Complications

01

Skeletonized appearance
A side effect of temporalis muscle injection with toxin can be a reduction in volume of the muscle, leading to a skeletonized appearance. Treatment consists of injecting volumizing fillers in the temporal area.

02

Hematoma
A number of arteries are found in the temporal area, including the superficial temporal artery, middle and deep temporal arteries, and periorbital venous plexuses. Avoidance can be improved by palpation. If an artery is inadvertently punctured, direct compression should be continued for at least 2 minutes in case of arterial puncture and 1 minute in case of venous puncture.

2.8 Lower eyelid wrinkles and widening of the eyes (orbicularis oculi muscle)

Injections must be placed very superficially and at a very low dose (0.5-1 U / 1.25-2.5 sU per injection, subcutaneously). In addition, hypertrophy of the pretarsal orbicularis oculi can be treated. 1-2 U lateral to the midpupillary line 1-2 mm below the lashes.

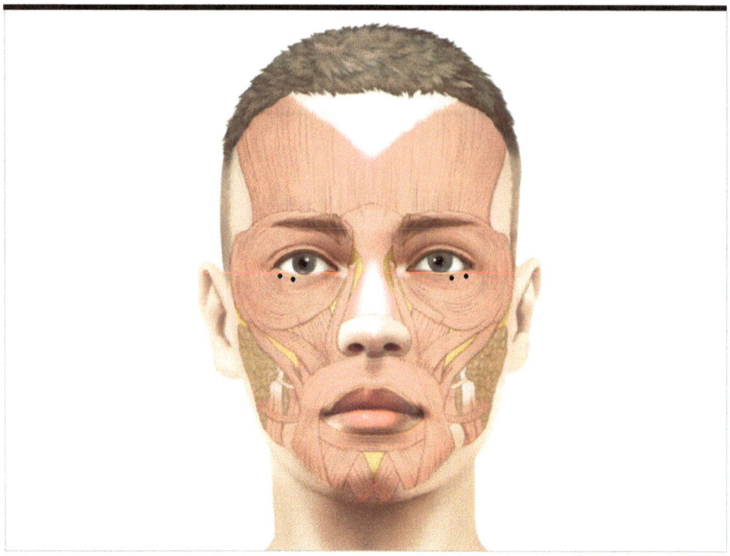

Figure 16
Injection pattern for treatment of the orbicularis oculi muscle

Toxin is administered at 1-2 injection points in the ramus tarsalis, 2-3 mm below the lashes with subcutaneous injection of 0.5-1 U / sU 1.25-2.5 per injection point. Injections are lateral to the midpupilliary line.

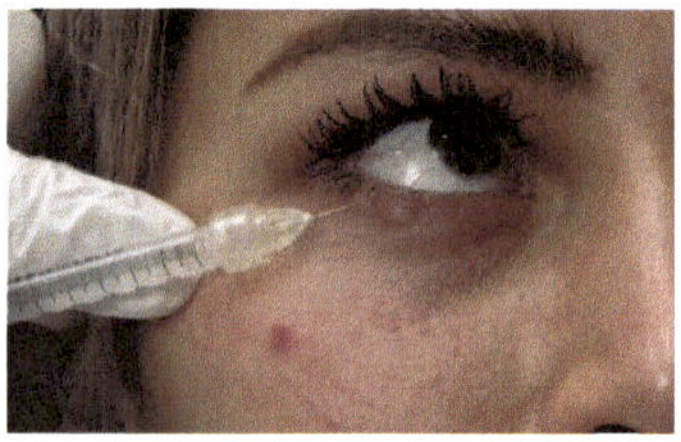

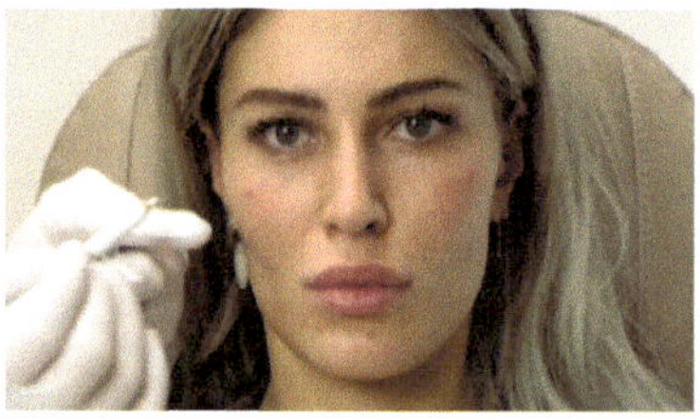

Figure 17 and Video 8
Lower eyelid wrinkles and widening of the eyes (orbicularis oculi muscle)

Two drops of 0.5U / 1.25 sU are injected subcutaneously in the lower eyelid while the patient is asked to look up.

Watch video at http://bit.ly/botulinum-toxin-in-aesthetic-medicine-uma-academy

Complications

01

Ectropion
Lower eyelid injection sites medial to the lateral canthus are associated with a higher risk of causing ectropion. Eyelid laxity must be tested prior to treatment by a snap test, which involves pulled down the lower eyelid with a finger and releasing. The eyelid should reposition (snap) quickly (within a second). A slow snap test indicates an increased risk for ectropion.

02

Eye bags
When the lower eyelids are treated, the tonus of the orbicularis oculi muscle may be weakened in such a way that it bulges anteriorly due to pressure of the underlying fat. To prevent this complication, the toxin dose for the lower eyelids should be limited to a maximum of 1 U / 2.5 sU per injection site. Infraorbital bags may also be caused by lymphatic stasis. The orbicularis oculi muscle has a pumping function for the drainage of lymphatic fluid. When this pump is weakened, stasis and accumulation of lymphatic fluid may result. This side effect can be prevented by minimizing the dose of toxin. It is self-limiting and usually disappears within 2 weeks as the lymphatic system adjusts to the new circumstances. Manual lymphatic drainage can help disperse the fluid.

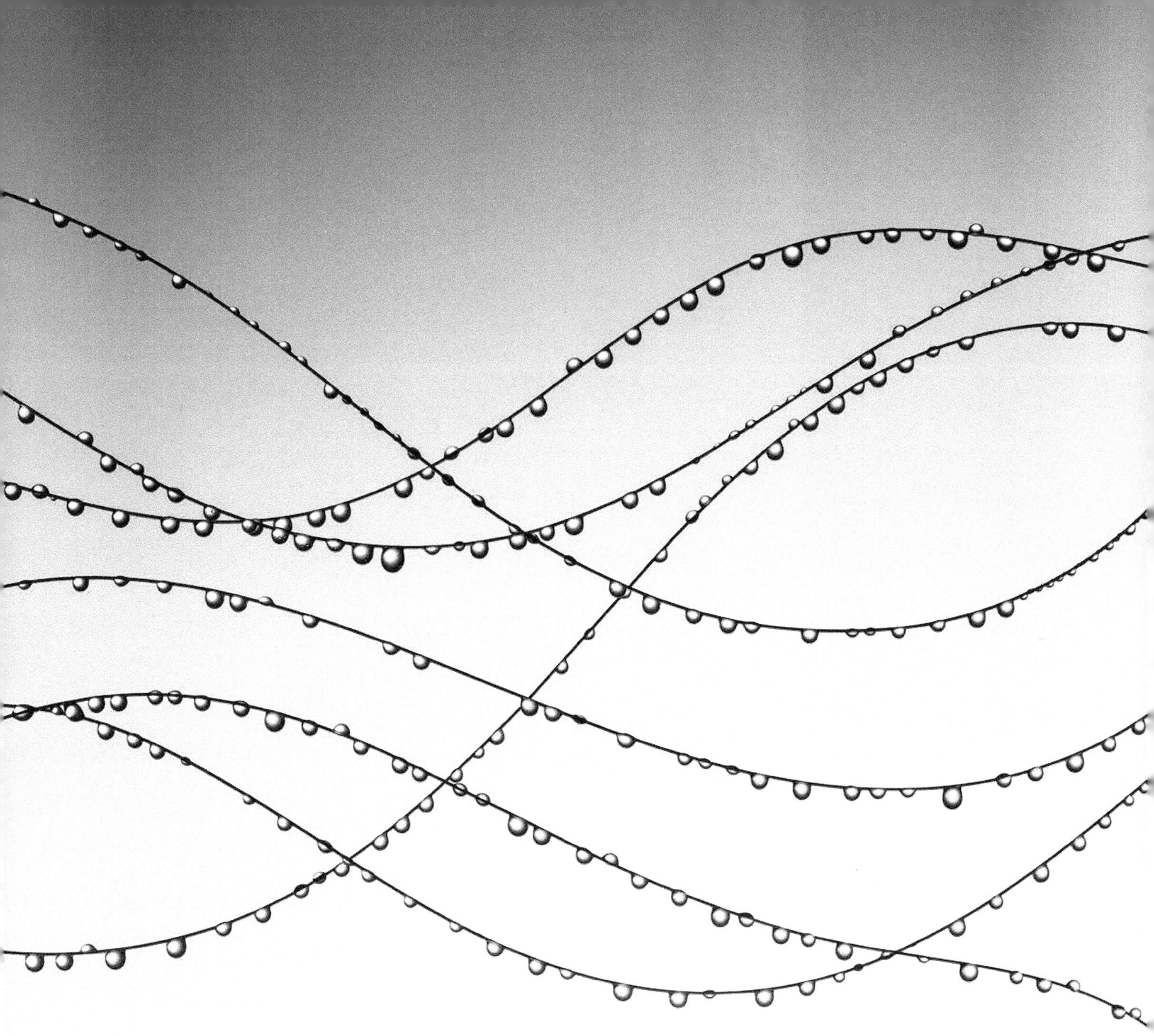

03

middle third of the face

introduction

Although the use of botulinum toxin is mainly indicated in the upper third of the face, there are several indications for the middle third of the face. These injections are more subtle and require more experience as an injector.

Proper knowledge of the anatomy and physiology of muscles is required. Especially around the modiolus, which has a complex equilibrium of agonistic and antagonistic actions of multiple muscles. Excessive or inappropriate injections lead to undesirable side effects. Adhering to the correct treatment protocols can lead to highly satisfying results, reducing bunny lines and peri-oral lines, correction of a gummy smile, and facial asymmetries.

middle third of the face

3.1 Bunny lines (LLSAN and depressor supercilii muscles)

Nasal rhytides or bunny lines can be treated by injecting 2-4 U / 5-10 sU of toxin at a depth of 2-4 mm, just above the center of the levator labii superioris aleque nasii muscle (LLSAN), and just medial to the vertical line between ala and medial canthus. At this position the muscle can be easily palpated during contraction. Concurrent treatment of the depressor supercilii muscle is sometimes also necessary in which case both sides should be injected with about 1-2 U / 2.5-5 sU at a depth of 1-2 mm injection pattern for nasal rhytides (bunny lines).

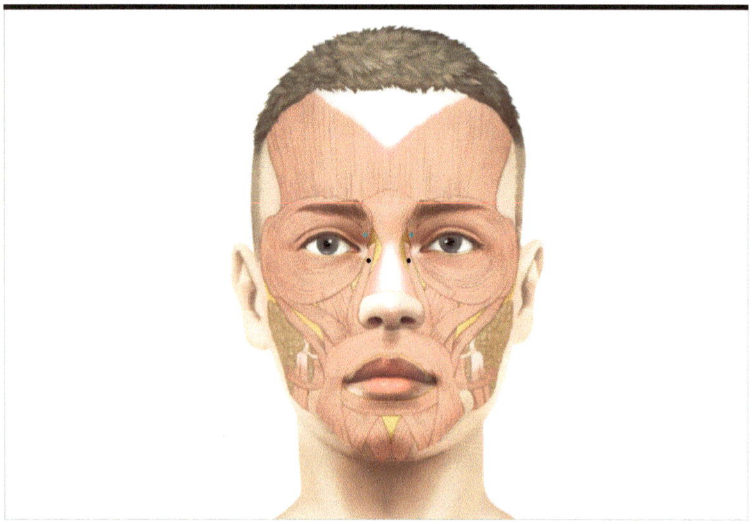

Figure 18
Injection pattern for nasal rhytides (bunny lines)

Black: the most common sites of injection (intramuscular injection technique) uses 2-4 U / 5-10 sU at an injection depth of 2-4 mm;
Blue: additional potential sites of injection intramuscularly 1-2 U / 2.5-5 sU, at a depth of 2-4 mm.

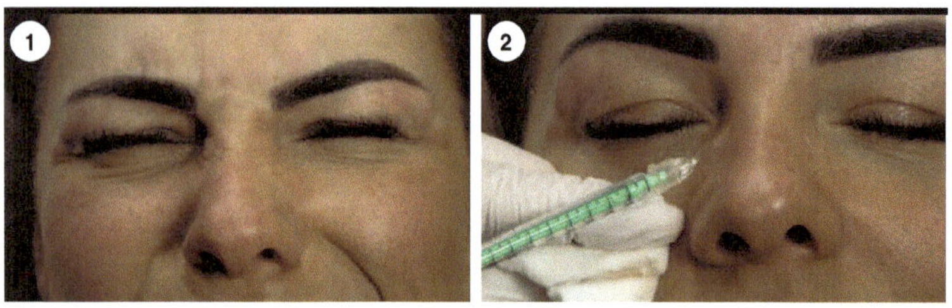

Figure 19
Bunny lines

1 Contract state
2 Markings and injection

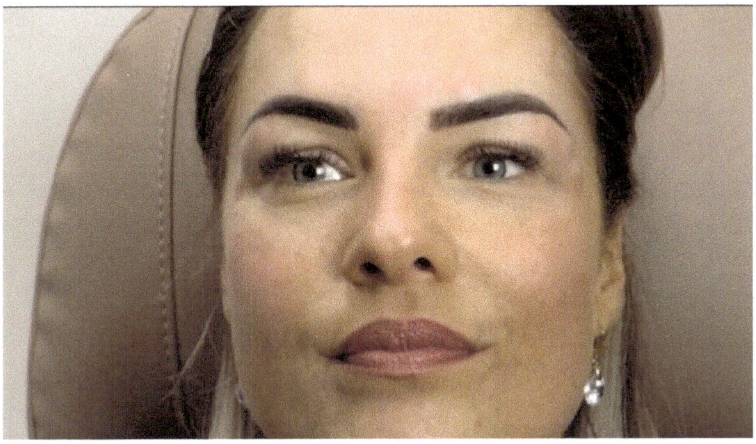

Watch video at http://bit.ly/botulinum-toxin-in-aesthetic-medicine-uma-academy

Video 9

Bunny lines

1. Glabellar complex in contracted state.
2. Markings and procerus muscle injection.
3. Deep injection in the medial side of the corrugator supercilii muscle.
4. Superficial injectio in the lateral side of the corrugator.

Complications

01

Altered smile

Injecting in the lower part of the LLSAN may lead to lowering of the upper lip and less visible teeth display when laughing. In order to prevent this side effect, inject cranial to the middle of the muscle, between the ala and medial canthus.

02

Diplopia

Unintentional treatment of the intraorbital muscles is a theoretical possibility with injection of the depressor supercilii muscle. Taking into account the diffusion radius, this complication can be prevented by keeping a distance of approximately 1 cm from the orbital rim.

03

Hematoma

The angular artery runs very close to the LLSAN. It is therefore wise to inspect the area well, as the artery is located subcutaneously. Care must also be taken with superior injection as the a. angularis runs close to the caudal insertion of the depressor supercilii muscle.

middle third of the face

3.2 Nasolabial fold and gummy smile (m. LLSAN and m. LLS)

A gummy smile can be treated by injection of 1-4 U / 2.5-10 sU of toxin in the inferior portion of the LLSAN, just above the top of the nasolabial fold, and next to the ala. The needle depth is 2-4 mm. Simultaneous treatment of the levator labii superioris (LLS) muscle is sometimes also necessary using 1-2 U / 2.5-5 sU at an injection depth of 1-2 mm, and at a maximum distance of 1 cm lateral to the ala.

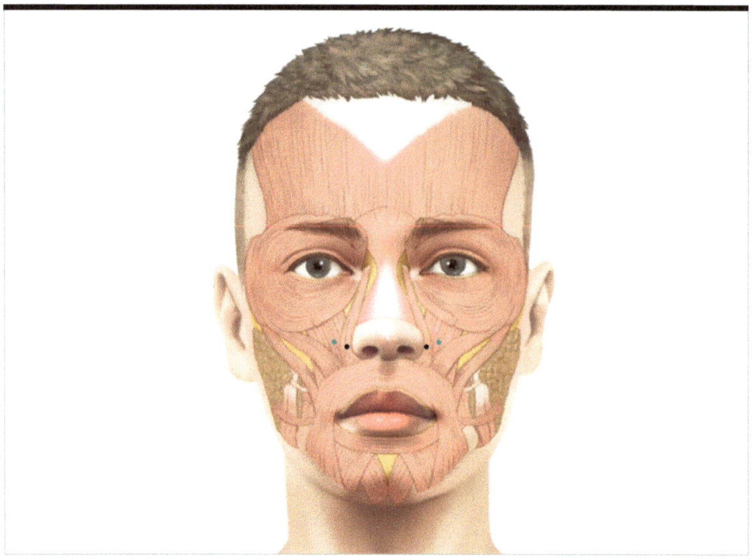

Figure 20
Injection pattern for treatment of visible gums when laughing or smiling and the nasallabial fold

Black: the most common sites of injection (intramuscular injection technique) using 1-4 U / 2.5-10 sU at an injection depth of 2-4 mm;
Blue: additional potential sites of injection (intramuscularly) using 1-2 U / 2.5-5 sU at an injection depth of 1-2 mm.

Complications

01

Altered smile
Although a change in smile is the purpose of this treatment, an unintended change in smile could also occur. Lateral to the LLS lies the zygomaticus minor muscle, a muscle that is important for smiling. The levator anguli oris lies deep to the LLS. This muscle is also important for the position of the oral commissure. To prevent a changed smile, the injection must therefore be very precise, as close as possible to the ala and superficial at a maximum injection depth of 2-3 mm.

02

Hematoma
The angular artery runs subcutaneously and parallel to the LLSAN. Due to its high degree of anatomic variation, there is always a possibility that this artery may be punctured. If a drop of blood is seen after the needle is removed, compress for a minute to prevent a large ecchymosis.

3.3 Perioral radial wrinkles (orbicularis oris muscle)

For the treatment of perioral lines, two injections are typically administered per quadrant as intradermal blebs of about 0.5-1 U / 1.25- 2.5 sU, 1-2 mm from the vermillion border. The injection depth is approximately 1-2 mm to prevent diffusion into the deeper LLSAN, levator anguli oris muscle (LAO) and zygomaticus minor muscle.

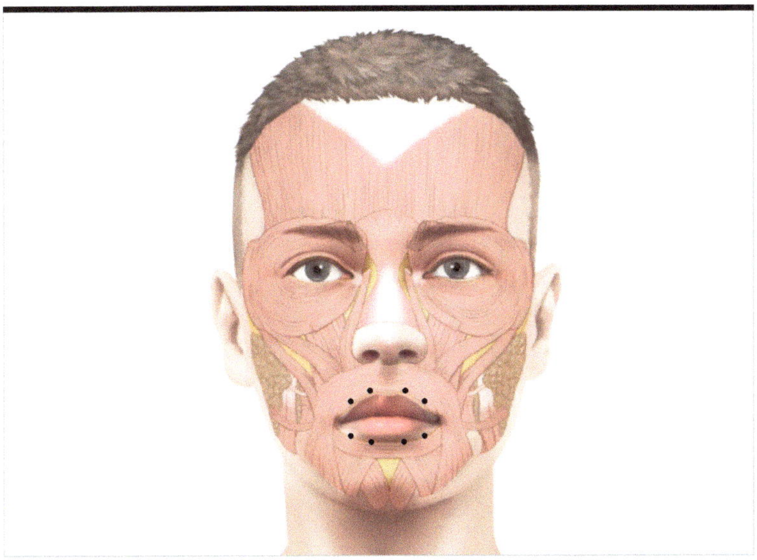

Figure 21
Injection pattern for radial perioral wrinkles

Black: the most common sites of injection (intradermal injection technique) using 0.5-1 U / 1.25-2.5 sU at an injection depth of 1-2 mm.

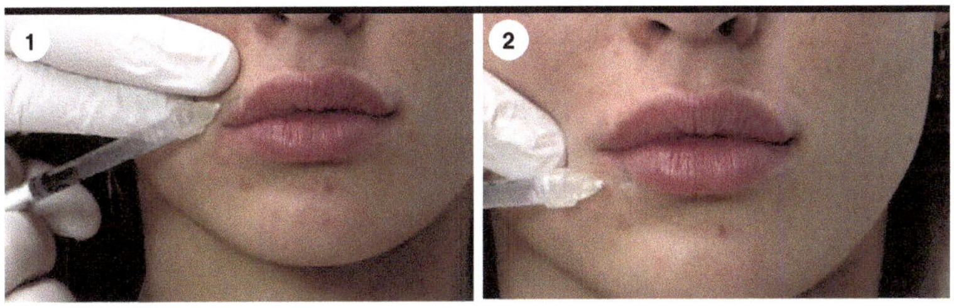

Figure 22
Treatment of the orbicularis oris for lip eversion

Each lip quadrant receives two injections, approximately 2mm from the vermillion border.
1 Upper lip
2 Lower lip

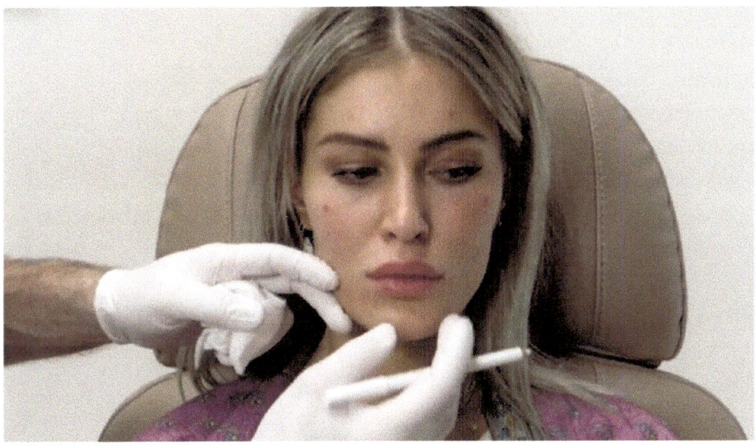

Watch video at http://bit.ly/botulinum-toxin-in-aesthetic-medicine-uma-academy

Video 10
Treatment of the orbicularis oris for lip eversion

Each lip quadrant receives two injections, approximately 2mm from the vermillion border.
1 Upper lip
2 Lower lip

middle third of the face

A low dose of botulinum toxin is warranted in order to prevent problems with eating, drinking and the pronounciation of certain letters.

Complications

01

Problems with eating and drinking
The orbicularis oris muscle is used to purse the lips, for example when drinking through a straw. Weakening of this muscle may therefore lead to unwanted restriction in normal eating and drinking movements. Pay attention to the dosage to prevent this complication; start low and titrate to the desired result.

02

Speaking problems
The orbicularis oris muscle is important for producing sounds, such as the letters p and b, as well as whistling. Botulinum toxin may reduce the ability of the muscle to produce these sounds. A low dosage is recommended to prevent this complication.

03

Hematoma
The superior labial artery runs submuscular laterally and becomes submuscular to medial superficially, with cranial branches. The presence of many vessels in this area means there is a risk of hematomas and injections should be superficial to reduce this risk.

04

Asymmetry
If the injection pattern is not symmetrical, asymmetry of the lip may result. It is therefore recommended to clearly mark the area to be treated before injecting.

05

Problems with lips and smile
When injection is performed too cranially and too deep, the botulinum toxin may affect the zygomaticus minor muscle, the levator labii superioris muscle (LLS) and LLSAN. Muscles attached to the modiolus may also be affected if injection is too lateral. Injection sites should therefore be close to the vermillion border and at least 1 cm medial to the oral commissure.

06

Inversion of the lower lip
When injection is too deep, botulinum toxin may affect the DLI which is located deep to the orbicularis oris muscle. It is therefore important to inject superficially.

3.4 Nose tip depression (depressor septi nasi muscle)

Before injecting ask the patient to smile to inspect the degree of depression and examine both laterally and anteriorly. Palpation of the nose tip during contraction can give an idea of the strength of the depressor septi nasi muscle. Mark the injection site in the middle of the columella or 1-2 mm closer to the nasal tip in order to prevent diffusion to the orbicularis oris muscle. Inject central in the middle of the columella as a single subdermal bolus of 2-4 U / 5-10 sU.

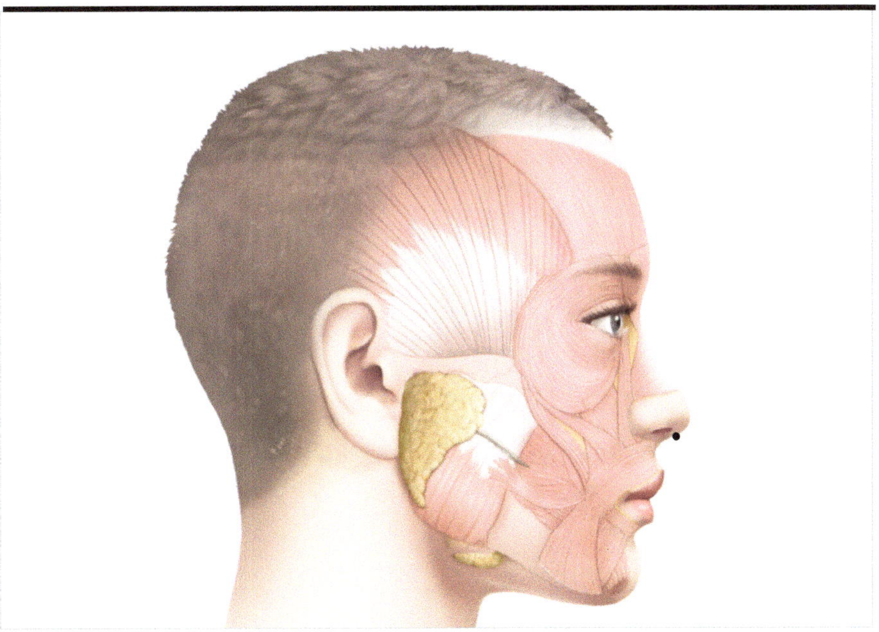

Figure 23
Injection pattern for nose tip depression (m. depressor septi nasi)

Inject the middle of the columella with a subdermal bolus of 2-4 U / 5-10 sU at an injection depth of 2-4 mm.

middle third of the face

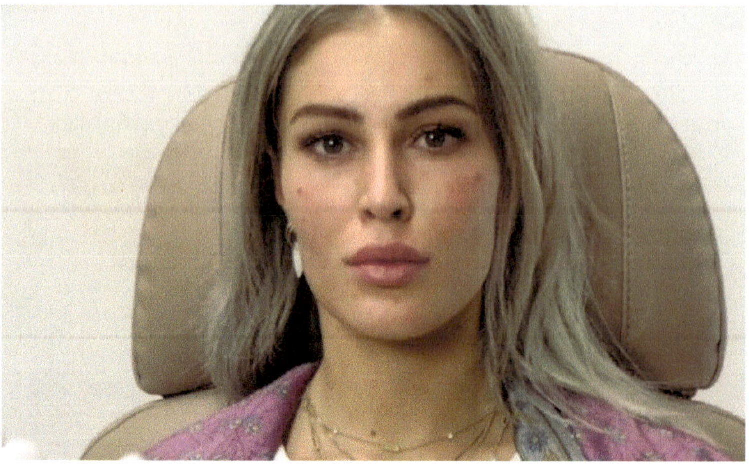

Watch video at http://bit.ly/botulinum-toxin-in-aesthetic-medicine-uma-academy

Video 11
Treatment of the m. depressor septi nasi

Treatment of depressor septi nasii muscle for nose tip elevation.

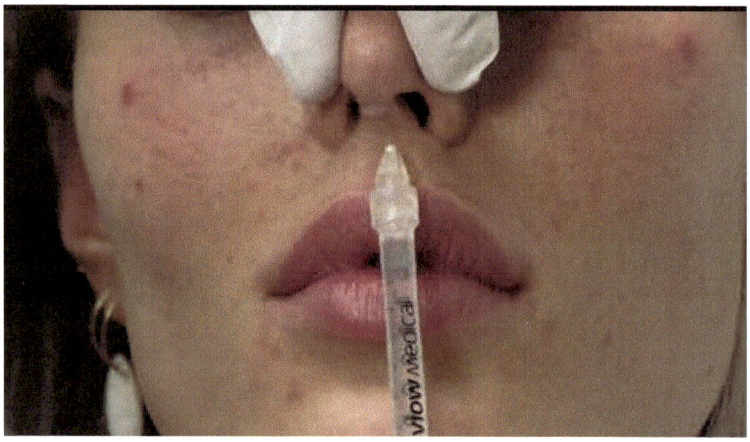

Figure 24
Treatment of the m. depressor septi nasi

Treatment of depressor septi nasii muscle for nose tip elevation.

Complications

01

Hematoma
Due to the proximity of the columellar artery, there is a risk of hematoma.

02

Weakness of the orbicularis oris muscle is a theoretical risk
To prevent this, the injection site should be closer to the nasal tip than the philtrum.

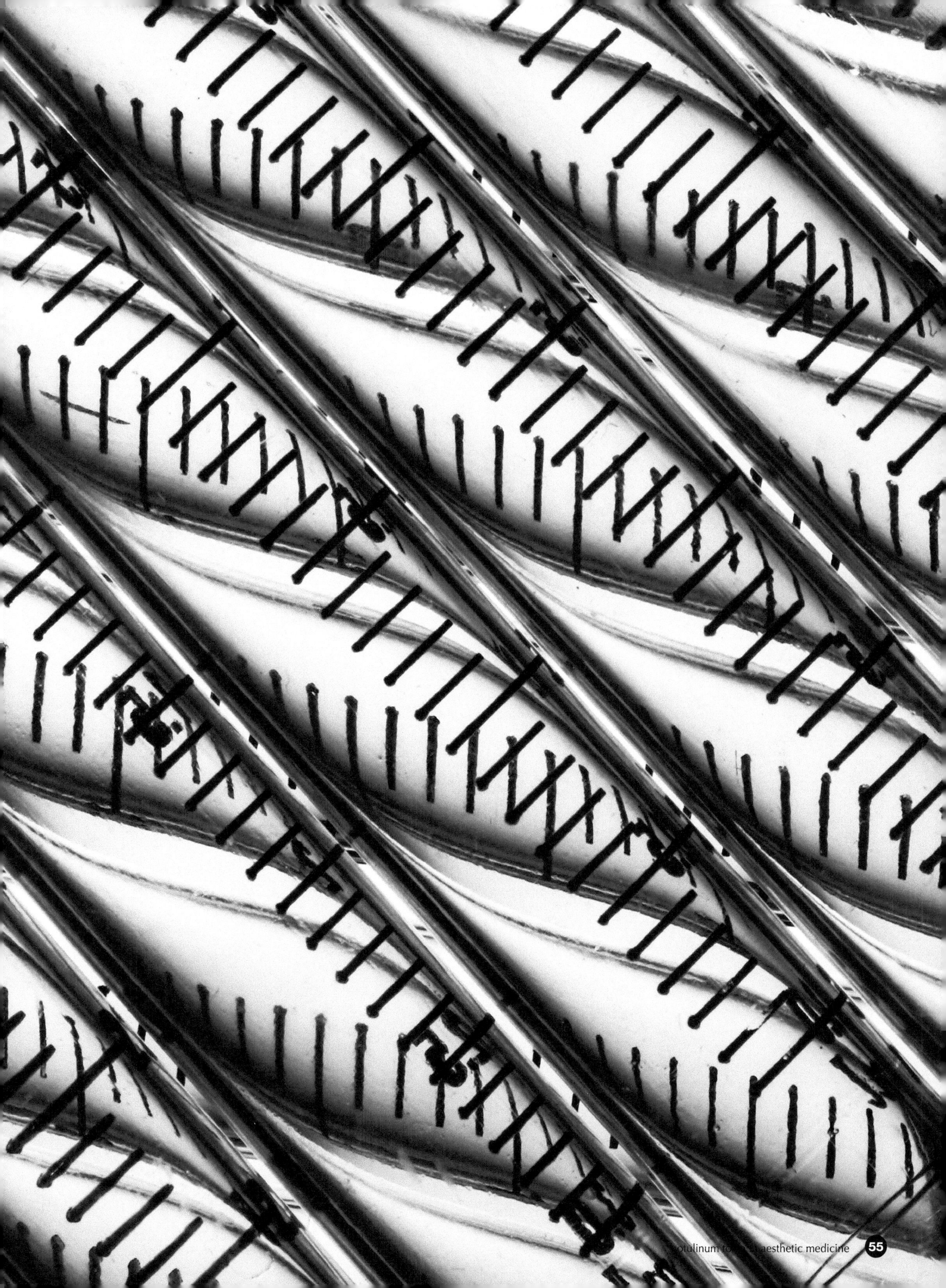

04
lower third of the face

introduction

The use of botulinum toxin in the lower third of the face is a popular way to rejuvenate the face. In this region, soft-tissue fillers usually are the first-line choice, rather than botulinum toxin, to provide structure and support. However, botulinum toxin can be considered for the treatment of dynamic lines, projection of the mentum, the mental crease, the position of the oral commissures, as well as for the treatment of hypertrophic masseter muscles which can lead to facial shape remodeling.

lower third of the face

4.1 Oral commissures (DAO)

The injection site is located mid-point between the oral commissures and the lower edge of the mandible, approximately 0.5 cm lateral to the Marionette line. Inject intramuscularly at a depth of 4-6 mm using 2-4 U / 5-10 sU. A possible second injection site is at the mandibular border. At this site, injection depth is 6-9 mm given the deep attachment to the marionette line pattern for a drooping mouth.

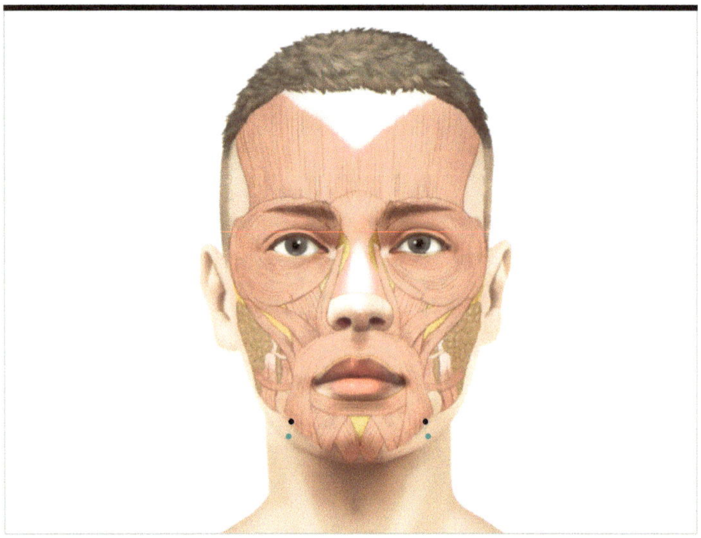

Figure 25
Injection pattern for a drooping mouth

Black: the most common sites of injection (intramuscular injection technique);
Blue: additional possible injection sites.

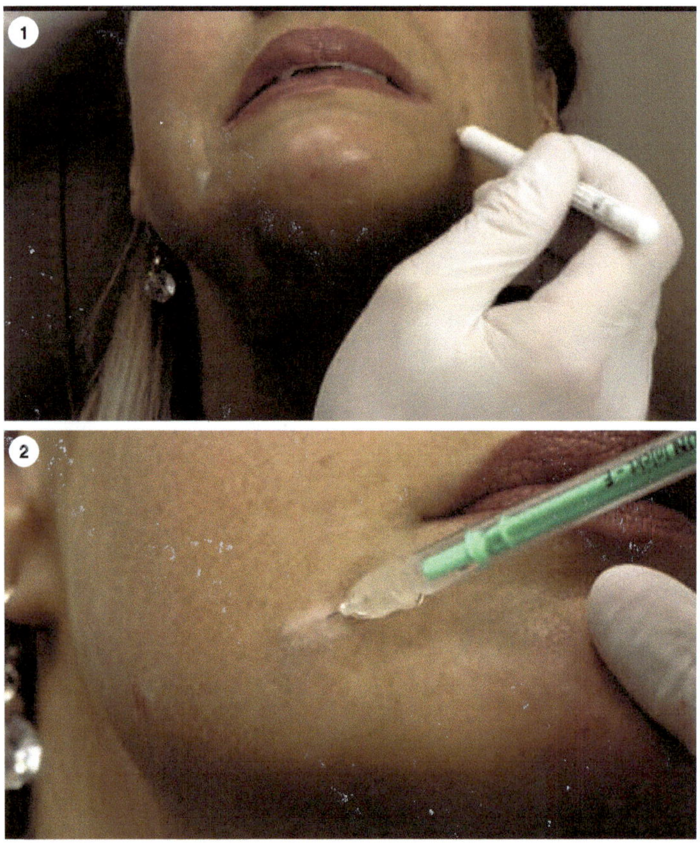

Figure 26
DAO injection

1 Contracted state of DAO and markings (if the muscle is difficult to see, the intersection point of a horizontal line at the middle of the distance between the oral commissure and the mandible with a line parallel to the nasolabial fold originating from the oral commissure can be used).
2 Injecting each marking with a superficial bolus and the needle directed towards the mandibular angle of the same side.

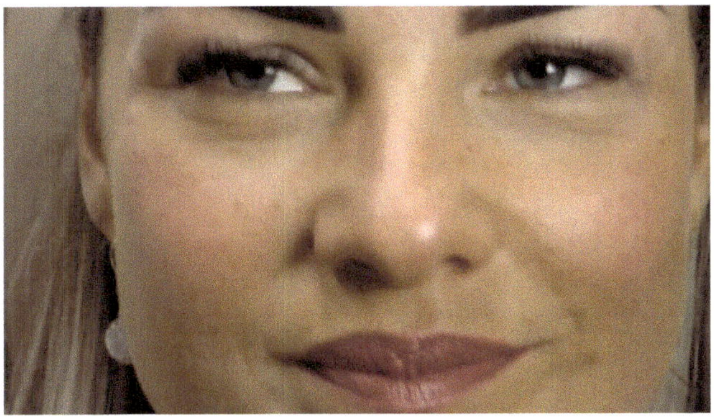

Watch video at http://bit.ly/botulinum-toxin-in-aesthetic-medicine-uma-academy

Video 12
DAO injection

Do not inject the botulinum toxin too medially to avoid the m. depressor labii inferioris which may result in a lower lip inversion.

Complications

01

Lower lip inversion
Inadvertent treatment of the depressor labii inferioris muscle (DLI) may cause the lower lip to invert because of the relatively increased pull of the orbicularis oris muscle. To prevent this side effect the injection site should not be placed too medially. A good way to achieve this is to direct the needle away from the DLI, in an inferolateral direction. Close to the mandibular border the DAO runs deep in relation to the DLI, and the latter can therefore be avoided by not injecting too superficially. Treatment of accidental DLI injection consists of weakening the orbicularis oris muscle on the same side: inject 1-2 U / 2.5-5 sU intradermally just below the vermillion border in the middle of the affected side of the lip.

02

Problems with eating
The DAO is used to move food from the cheek to the tongue and when weakened can make eating difficult. Prevention is by avoiding high doses; treatment is expectative.

03

Speaking problems
Injecting too cranially in the area of the modiolus can affect the orbicularis oris muscle. As this muscle is important for pronouncing certain sounds, its weakening may lead to speech problems. Prevention is by avoiding injections near the lip; treatment is expectative.

04

Hematoma
The facial artery runs lateral to the DAO and hematoma can result if injections are performed too laterally. The inferior labial artery runs deep in relation to the DAO and deep injections in this area should therefore be avoided. Treatment of hematoma consists of direct pressure.

lower third of the face

4.2 Mental crease and mentalis dimples (mentalis muscle)

The chin is treated with a bilateral injection in the belly of the mentalis muscle using 2-6 U / 5-15 sU of toxin. The injections are located 1-3 mm from the midline at a depth of approximately 4-9 mm to prevent diffusion to the laterally- and more superficially-located DLI. The cranial area of the muscle does not require treatment to reduce the risk of spread to the orbicularis oris muscle. Injection pattern for chin dimples and horizontal sulcus (mental crease).

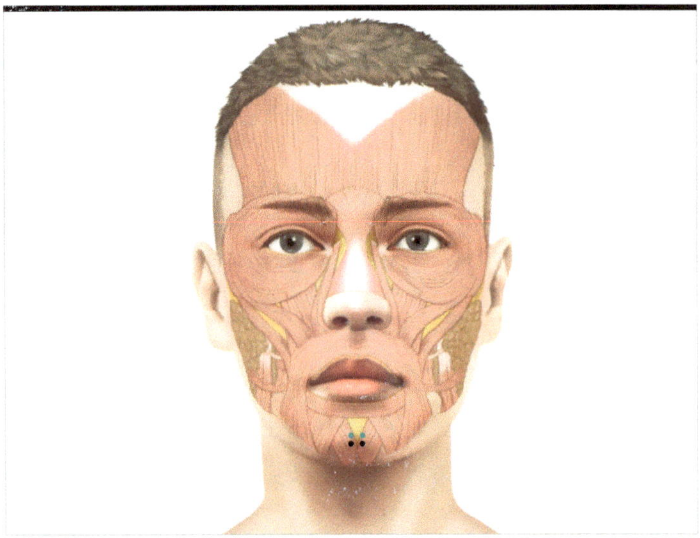

Figure 27
Injection pattern for chin dimples and horizontal sulcus (mental crease)

Black: the most common injection sites (deep intramuscular injection technique) using 2-6 U / 5-15 sU
Blue: additional potential injection sites, intramuscular.

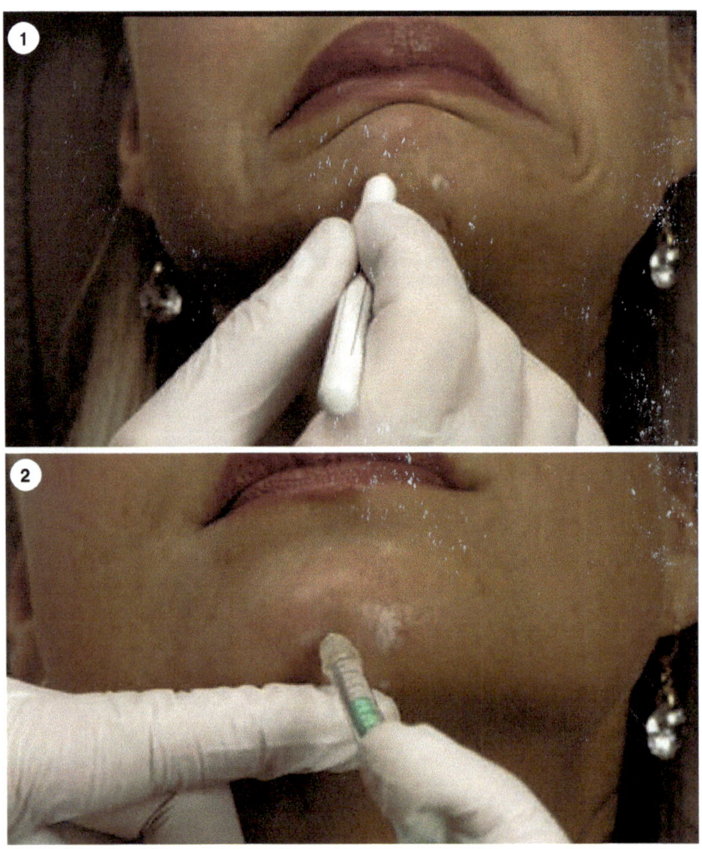

Figure 28
Mentalis injection

1 Contracted state of mentalis muscle (pouting lower lip). Marking at the dimples that indicate skin insertions.
2 Injecting each marking with a deep bolus.

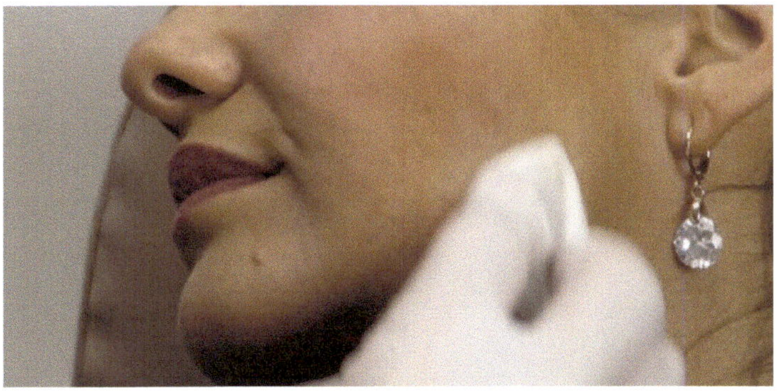

Video 13
Mentalis injection

Watch video at http://bit.ly/botulinum-toxin-in-aesthetic-medicine-uma-academy

Complications

01

Inversion of the lower lip
This can occur when the DLI is unintentionally treated. To avoid this undesirable effect, botulinum toxin should be injected deep into the mentalis muscle as the DLI is more superficial. Moreover, injections should be medial as the DLI is situated lateral to the mentalis muscle. If the DLI is affected, small doses of 1-2 U / 2.5-5 sU should be injected in the orbicularis oris muscle.

lower third of the face

4.3 Masseter hypertrophy (masseter muscle)

To determine masseter hypertrophy (MH) the patient is asked to clench their jaw/teeth as the masseter muscle can then be easily palpated. With the jaws clenched, the ends of the muscle can be determined for the second and third injection. The published total dosage varies from 12 U / 30 sU to 56 U / 140 sU per side. As a standard, we recommend an average dosage of 40 U / 100 sU divided over six injections (3 per side) with the central injection having half the dose per side and the other two having 25% of the dose each. The cranial limit of the treatment area is an imaginary line from the earlobe to the oral commissure. The treatment area should also stop 1.5 cm from the end of the muscle to prevent complications due to spreading or diffusion to other muscles. The effect on volume reduction will take longer than the time required for the muscle to weaken. The muscle strength decreases in 2 weeks, but the improvement in contour will take longer.

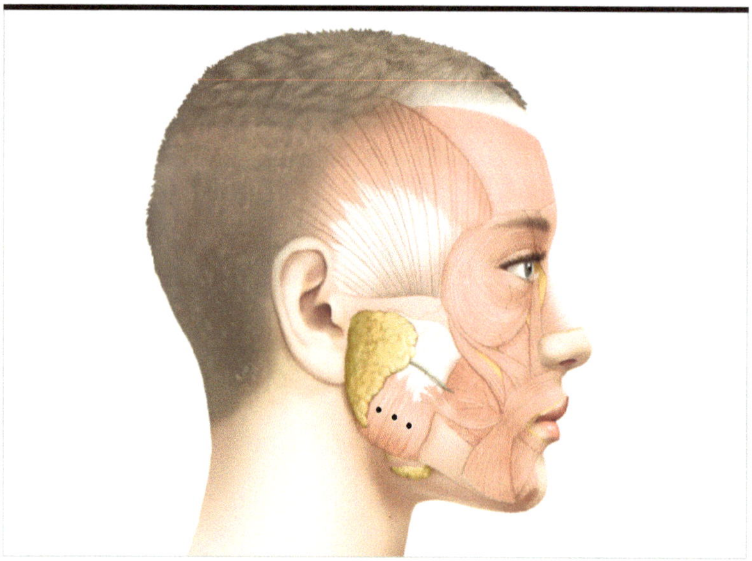

Figure 29
Injection pattern for masseter hypertrophy (masseter muscle)

In the middle of the muscle belly inject an intramuscular retrograde bolus of 10 U / 25 sU (middle black dot) at a depth of approximately 13 mm. Due to the retrograde injection of the toxin, the superficial muscle compartment should be reached. Two additional intramuscular boluses of 5 U / 7.5 sU are then injected 2 cm to either side of the first injection point at a depth of 10 mm.

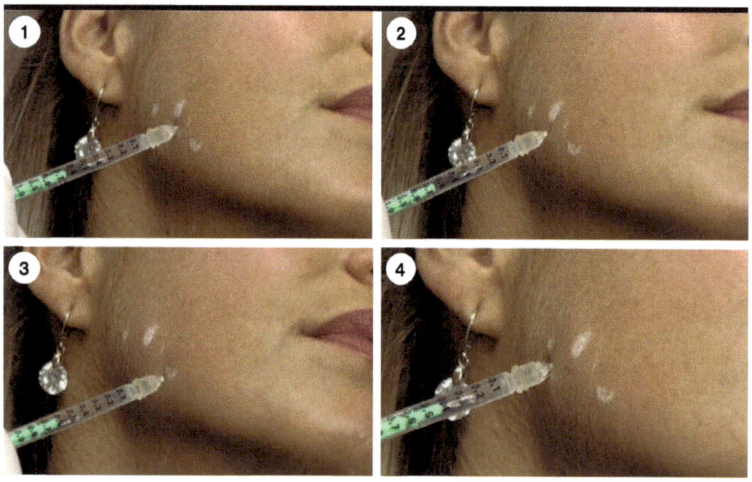

Figure 30
Masseter injection

1 Central masseter belly receives 50% of the dose, of which 75% deep.
2 25% of the central masseter dose is injected into the superficial masseter compartment.
3 The anterior masseter receives 25% of the total dose.
4 The posterior masseter also receives 25% of the total dose.

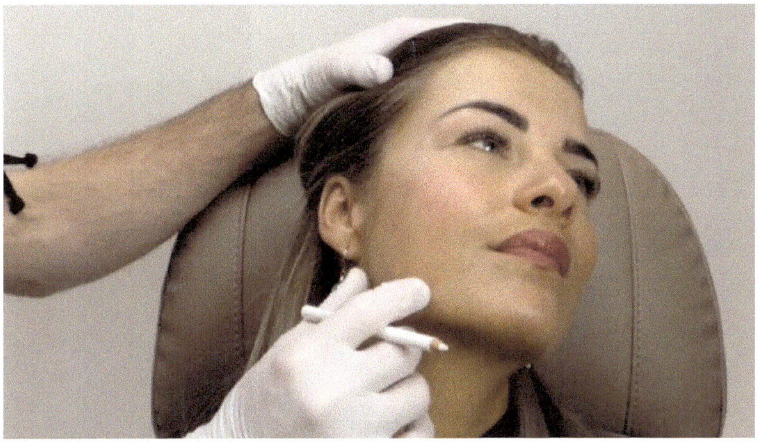

Watch video at http://bit.ly/botulinum-toxin-in-aesthetic-medicine-uma-academy

Video 14
Masseter injection

Complications with masseter hypertrophy

01

Paradoxical masseteric bulging
A deep inferior tendon (DIT) structure separates the superficial belly from the deep muscle fibers. When only deep injection is performed, the superficial muscle compartment remains unaffected and a reactive hypercontraction of the superficial masseter belly can occur. Prevention is by injecting in the superficial compartment by using a retrograde injection technique. Treatment consists of injecting additional toxin to the superficial compartment.

02

Drooping mouth
By affecting the cranially located zygomaticus major muscle the corners of the mouth can droop and the smile may be altered. To prevent this, the injections should be limited to the lower half of the masseter muscle; caudal to the line between the oral commissure and the earlobe.

03

Altered smile
In addition to influencing the zygomaticus major muscle, the superficially located risorius muscle can be affected. To prevent this, the injection should be deep into the muscle (3/4 to full needle depth), particularly the medial injection.

04

Weakness when chewing
High doses can result in the masseter becoming so weak that the patient will notice an effect when chewing, especially when the temporalis muscle is also injected.

Treatment of the m. masseter can be used to slim down the lower third of the face, but can also be used for treatment of bruxism.

4.4 Jawline lift (platysma muscle and DAO)

With this treatment the downward force of the platysma muscle and the DAO will be reduced, which has an effect on the position of the skin at the jawline. The treatment protocol for the DAO is followed, with the addition of three injections into the platysma muscle.

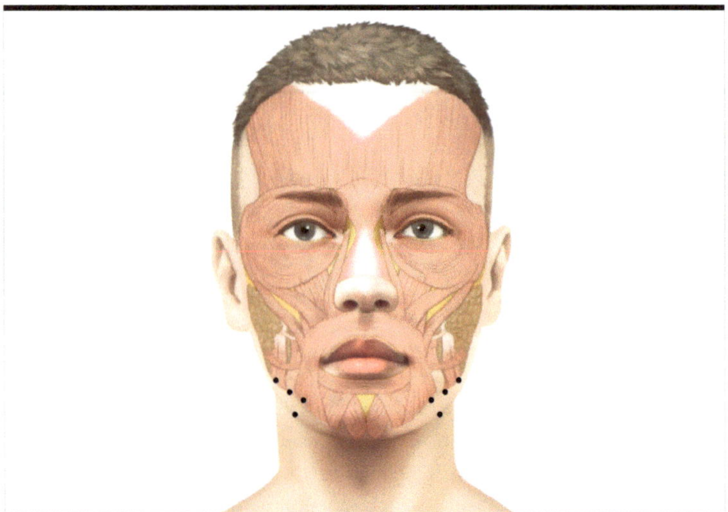

Figure 31
Jawline lift

Inject the DAO with an intramuscular bolus technique 2-4 U / 5-10 sU per injection. Then inject 2 cm lateral in platysma muscle with an intramuscular bolus technique 2-4 U / 5-10 sU and about 2 cm lateral again. A final injection using an intramuscular bolus technique and 2-4 U / 5-10 sU is placed in the anterior submental muscle bundle of the platysma muscle directly under the mandible.

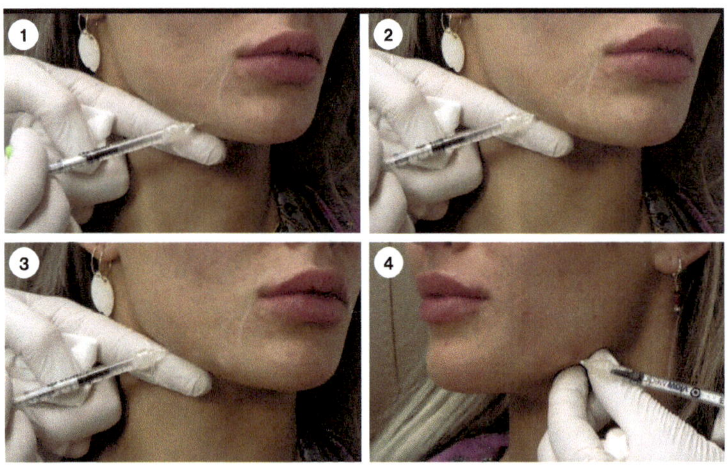

Figure 32
Jawline lift

1
DAO injection.
2, 3, 4
Platysma injection.

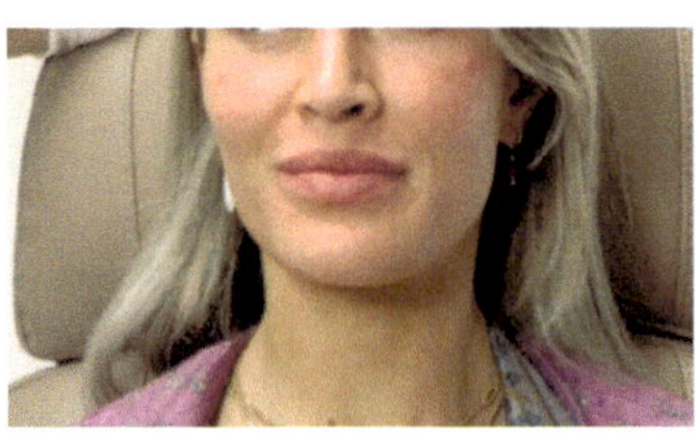

Video 15
Jawline lift

1 DAO injection.
2 Platysma injection.

Watch video at http://bit.ly/botulinum-toxin-in-aesthetic-medicine-uma-academy

Complications

Complications are the same as for the DAO (see Lower Third of the Face, chapter 4).

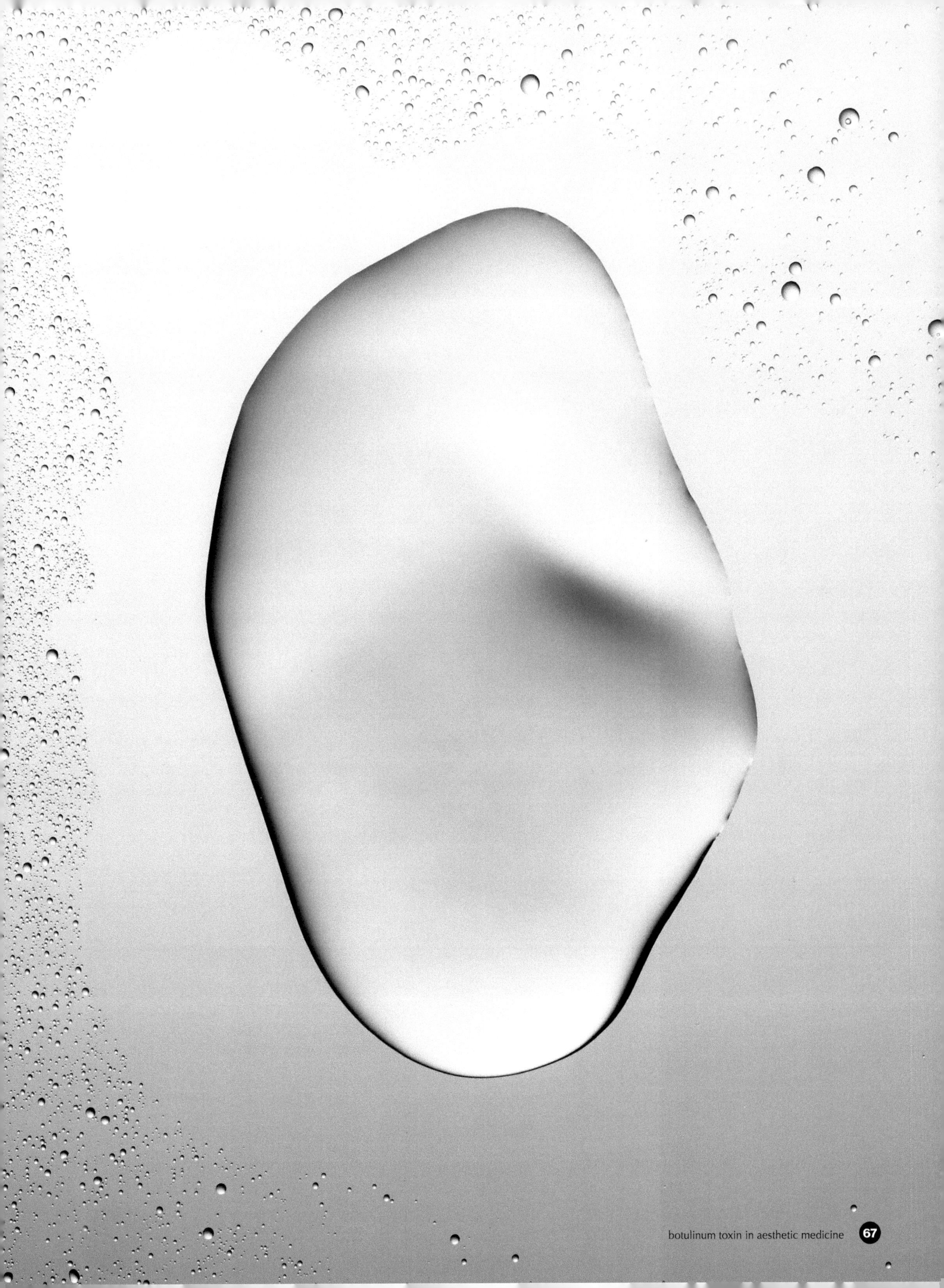

05

non-facial indications

introduction

Although many areas of the body often require multiple treatment modalities for optimal rejuvenation, botulinum toxin can aid in muscle relaxation (e.g., platysma muscle) or primary focal hyperhidrosis. Excessive sweating can have a major impact on quality of life of the patient, resulting in social and work impairment. The aesthetic results for the patient is that they no longer have sweat stains in their clothes and an increase in self-confidence.

non-facial indications

5.1 Vertical muscle bands in the neck and horizontal neck lines

Platysmal bands

The platysmal bands are visualized by asking the patient to flex the platysma by clenching their teeth and pulling the corners of their mouth downward. The platysmal band is taken between the thumb and index finger of the non-dominant hand and a series of injections placed in the muscle bundles from the mandible to the clavicle as necessary. Injections of 2 U / 5sU with a maximum dose of 40 U / 100 sU per side are given intramuscularly with a distance of approximately 2 cm between the injection sites. The skin and subcutaneous fat in this area are very thin so subdermal injection will also be effective.

Horizontal neck creases

When treating horizontal necklines, the fibers of platysma that insert into the skin will be relaxed. Inject the wrinkles intradermally with 3-4 injection sites per side using 1-2 U / 2.5-5 sU of toxin at an injection depth of approximately 2 mm, and spacing the injections approximately 1-2 cm apart.

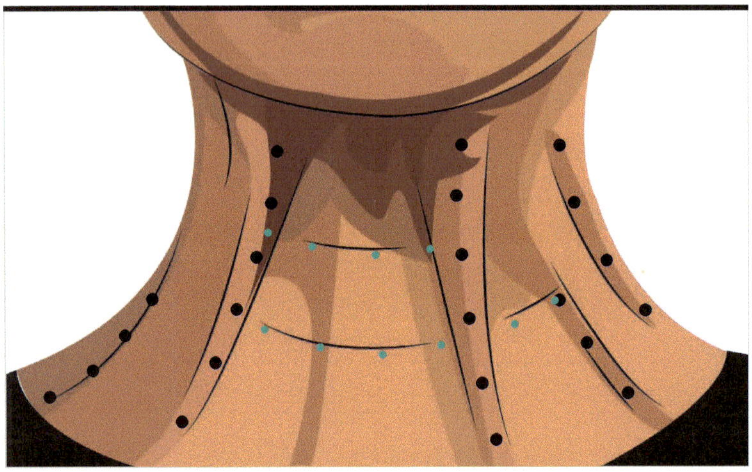

Figure 33

Injection pattern of the platysmal bands

Black dots: injection pattern for vertical muscles in the neck (platysma muscle bands). Mark the injection sites of the muscle bundles every 2 cm in the flexed state. Injections are performed in a relaxed state with a subdermal or intramuscular bolus technique using 2 U / 5 sU per injection.

Blue dots: injection pattern for horizontal creases in the neck (platysma muscle). Inject every 0.5-1 cm with an intradermal bolus technique using 0.5-1 U / 1.25-2.5 sU per injection site. The maximum dosage for treatment of the platysma muscle is 40 U / 100 sU per side. Image acquired from Ascher B, et al. JEADV 2010;24(11):1285-1295 and edited.

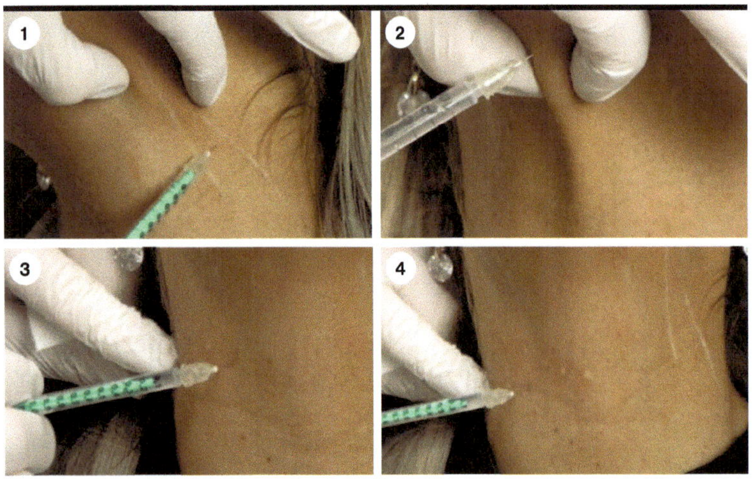

Figure 34

Vertical muscle bands in the neck and horizontal neck lines

1 Mark the platysma bands. Ask the patient to clench the teeth and pull the corners of the mouth downward.

2 Fixate the muscle between thumb and index finger and inject intramuscular.

3 and **4** Intradermal injections of the visual horizontal neck lines will help to relax them.

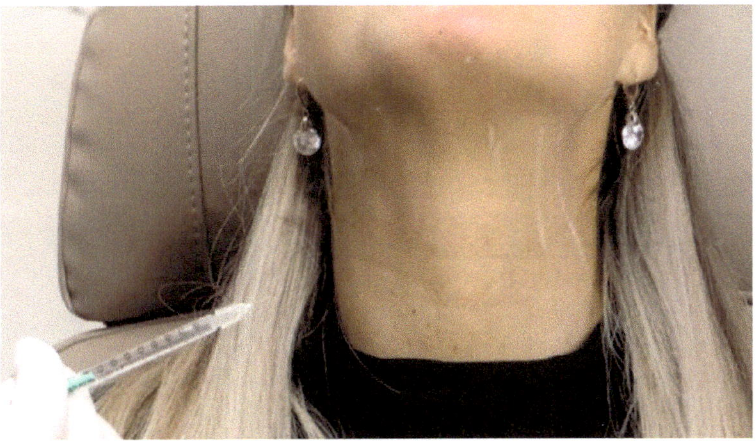

Watch video at http://bit.ly/botulinum-toxin-in-aesthetic-medicine-uma-academy

Video 16
Platysma injection

1 Contracted state of platysma and markings.
2 Injecting each platysma band with intramuscular boluses 2 cm apart while holding the band between the fingers of the non-dominant hand.
3 Injecting intradermal blebs of approximately 0.5 U / 1.25 sU into the horizontal neck lines.

Complications with platysma injections

01

Difficulty with swallowing or speaking
May occur with high doses and deep injection due to diffusion to the vocal cords and deeper muscles. To avoid this, injections should be superficial and in low doses (maximum of 40 U / 100 sU per side in the neck) spread over several injection sites for a good distribution of toxin. High-dose boluses should be avoided in proximity to the vocal chords to reduce the risk of spread to deeper muscles in the area.

02

Hematoma
The facial artery and the jugular vein run directly under the platysma muscle. Hematomas can therefore be avoided by ensuring injections are superficial.

non-facial indications

5.2 Primary focal hyperhidrosis

Primary hyperhidrosis is a chronic idiopathic condition associated with excessive sweating in the armpits, palms, soles and/or face. Botulinum toxin has a blocking effect on eccrine sweat glands as well as apocrine (cholinergic) glands.
It is one of the most common treatments for hyperhidrosis, with a low risk of side effects and high patient satisfaction. The desired aesthetic result is to prevent visible wet patches on clothing, and moist skin or sweaty hands.
With the iodine-starch test the hyperhidrotic surface of the axilla is easily made visible. An alternative (less messy) method to determine the area to inject uses the "pen slide test". With this method the shaved axilla if first degreased with alcohol. After several minutes, the alcohol will have evaporated and the skin will be dry. The pen will now slide smoothly over the dry skin. When the pen reaches the hyperhidrotic skin surface, the sweat will make the skin sticky and prevent the pen from sliding further. The limit of the hyperhidrotic area is then marked and divided into grid of 1 cm wide squares. Injections of 50-100 U / 125-250 sU distributed evenly throughout the squares are administered using an intradermal bleb injection technique.

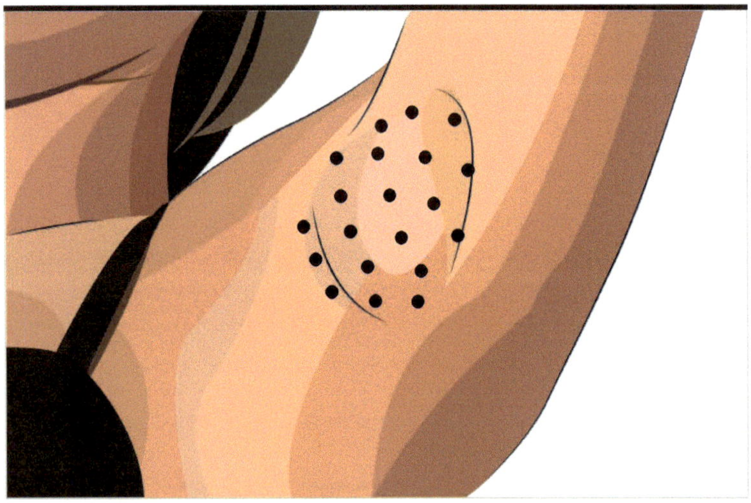

Figure 35

Primary focal hyperhidrosis

After marking a general treatment area, via the alcohol-pencil test, evenly distribute the product with intradermal injections.

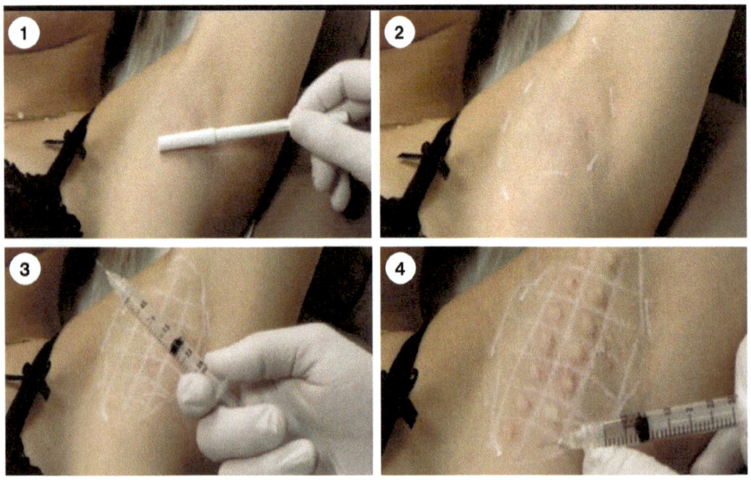

Figure 36

Primary focal hyperhidrosis

1, 2 As an alternative for the iodine-starch test, we use the alcohol-pen slide test to mark the treatment area.
3 Reconstitution of 50U/125sU in 2ml sodium chloride.
4 Evenly distribute the toxin over the treatment area.

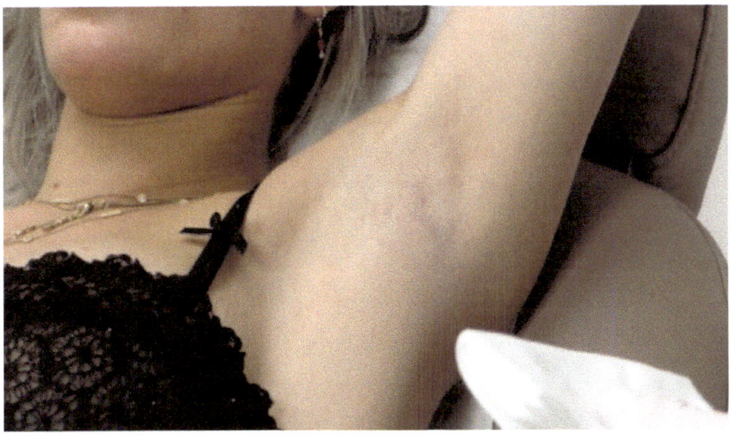

Watch video at http://bit.ly/botulinum-toxin-in-aesthetic-medicine-uma-academy

Video 17

Treating axillary hyperhidrosis

1. To determine the area of excessive perspiration, the axillae are disinfected with alcohol 70%. After the skin has had the opportunity to dry, the area with higher perspiration will become moist. Sliding a pen or cap over the dry skin will stop when the skin is moist.
2. All intersections between dry and wet skin are marked.
3. A grid of approximately 1x1 cm squares is drawn.
4. After counting the number of squares, 2 ml (50 U / 125 sU) per axilla is injected in even deposits at the dermal level.

5.3 Palmar and plantar hyperhidrosis

The palm or sole is first anesthetized with application of ice, anaesthetic creme or ulnar and radial nerve block. A grid of 2x2 cm squares is then marked and toxin injected subcutaneously in the center of each square for a total amount of 100 U / 250 sU per palm or sole. Side effects of the treatment are injection site pain and sometimes temporary weakness of the intrinsic hand or foot muscles.

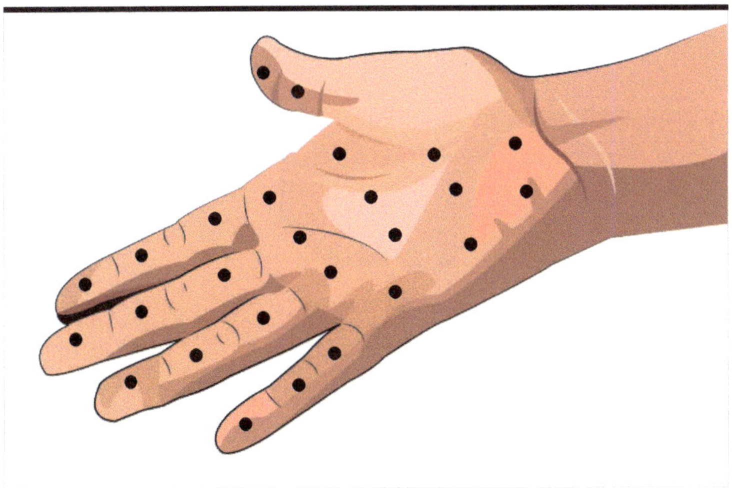

Figure 37

Markings for the intradermal injection technique in the palm of the hand.

The same principle will hold for the sole of the feet.

non-facial indications

5.4 Calf shaping with botulinum toxin

Botulinum neurotoxin has been used for improving body contours. Especially in Asia, many body indications have been explored, including the shoulders (deltoid muscle), neck (trapezius muscle) and lower legs (gastrocnemius muscle). Especially the latter has international interest in patients seeking a more slender appearance of their calf muscles. Depending on the desired reduction of volume, typically 40-100 U (100-250 sU) are injected in either the medial or lateral head of the gastrocnemius belly, using 2-4 U (5-10 sU) intramuscular injection points approximately 1 cm apart.

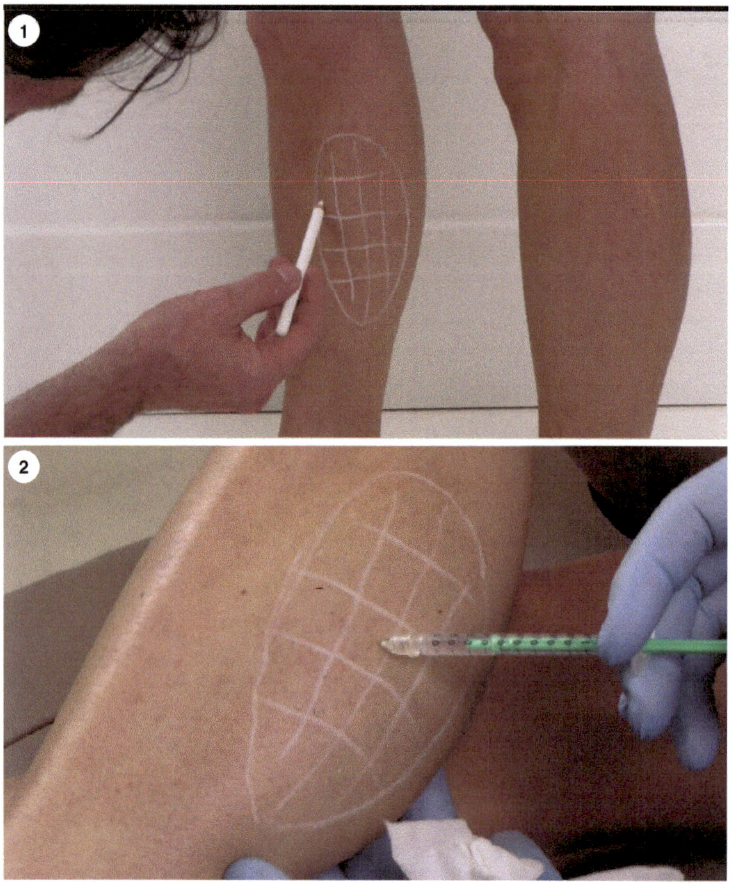

Figure 38
Calves

1 Mark the area that should be reduced in projection (either medial or lateral gastrocnemius, or both). Mark 1x1 squares.
2 Inject 2-4 U (5-10 sU) per square intramuscularly

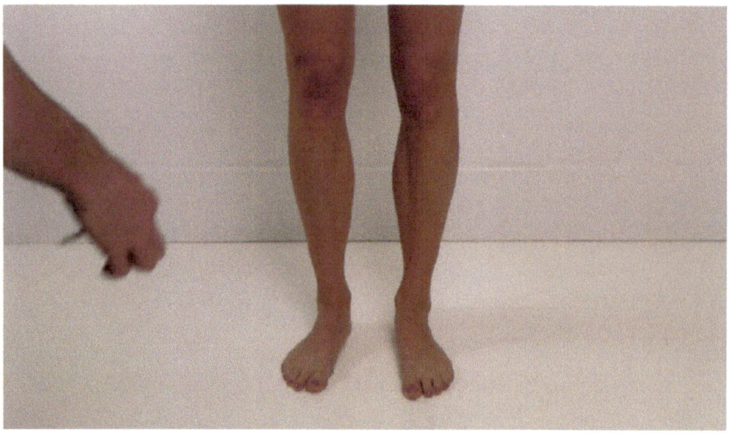

Video 18
Calves

After reconstitution of the botulinum toxin product according to the manufacturer's instructions for use, intramuscular injections are applied in the muscular area to be reduced in volume. The apex of the muscle may be injected with additional points as needed, like is shown in this video.

Watch video at http://bit.ly/botulinum-toxin-in-aesthetic-medicine-uma-academy

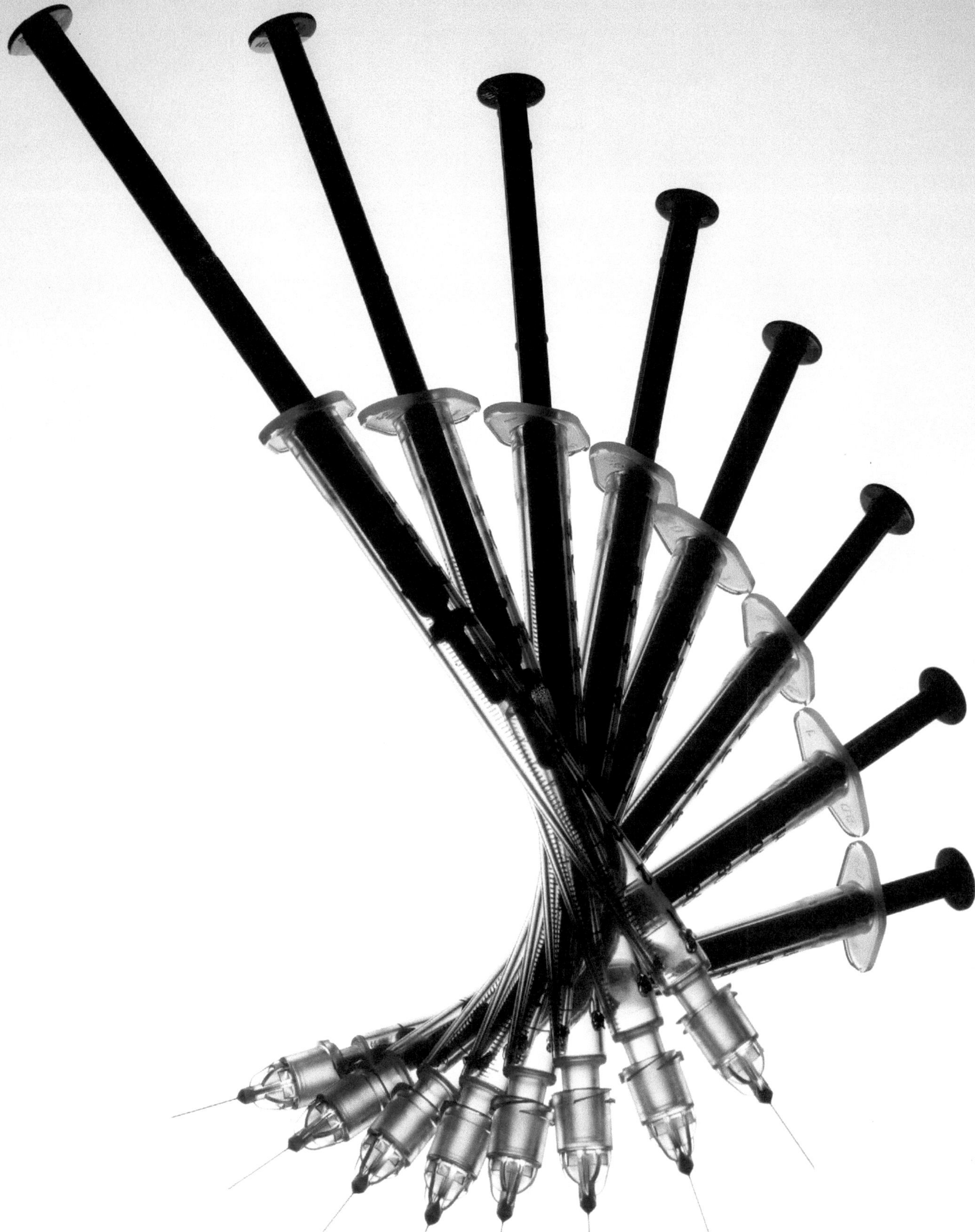

06
skin quality improvement with botulinum toxin

introduction

As the amount of indications for botulinum toxin is increasing yearly, a separate section is now in order focusing on novel observations on aesthetic improvement of the facial skin. As we know, hyperhidrosis can be treated because of the effects botulinum toxin has on the sweat glands. But also sebum secretion is affected and direct stimulation of fibroblasts is suggested after in-vitro study observations. Therefore, clinical effects have been reported on hydration, erythema, scarring, sebum production and pore count. In this chapter, we discuss the effects of botulinum toxin with specific reconstitution ratio on lifting the face with a so-called microtoxin treatment protocol and we also cover its effects on androgenetic alopecia. For all these skin quality improving procedures step by step protocols are supplied.

treatment of abnormal scarring

6.1. Botulinum toxin for the treatment of abnormal scarring

Wound healing is a complex phenomenon that includes a variety of physiologic responses to injury to the different organs, commonly the skin. The normal wound healing occurs in three overlapping, but biologically distinct, phases. The inflammatory phase starts immediately after the injury. Its purpose is to remove devitalized tissue and prevent infection. The proliferative phase is when granulation tissue fills the wound and keratinocytes migrate to restore epithelial continuity. Finally, the remodeling phase maximizes the strength and structural integrity of the wound.

Just as with everything else, wound healing can be impaired. Abnormal scarring usually is classified as either hypertrophic scarring or keloid formation. Histologically, hypertrophic scars and keloids are different. Keloids are characterized by the overgrowth of dense fibrous tissue beyond the borders of the original wound, as opposed to hypertrophic scars, where the overgrowth stays within the borders of the wound. Keloids are composed of closely packed fibrils and are more likely to produce dysfunctional contractures, impacting the patient's quality of life.

To date, there is no golden standard for treating hypertrophic scars and keloids. Limited understanding of the complex processes that occur in scar formation is the base of the lack of creating a golden standard. Intralesional injection with a corticosteroid is the most often chosen therapy but causes adverse events such as pain and pruritus. Alternatively, botulinum toxin type A can be injected. Botulinum toxin can relieve wound tension by relaxing the surrounding muscles. Besides, it may modulate fibroblasts causing inhibition of activity.[27-32] Both tissue tension and overactive fibroblast proliferation are considered key factor in keloid formation. Compared with corticosteroids, a recently published meta-analysis concluded that botulinum toxin is more effective and had a lower adverse events rate.[33] However, bias was introduced as most endpoints were subjective scales. Also, the included studies were mainly conducted in the Asian population, while African ethnicities are more likely to form keloids. Other shortcomings are the short follow up periods and the variation in the treatment regimens. Further studies need to be executed to evaluate the efficacy and most optimal treatment regimen of botulinum toxin for the treatment of abnormal scarring in all ethnicities.

Treatment of hypertrophic and keloid scars with botulinum neurotoxin type A.
The following step-by-step protocol can be used for treating hypertrophic and keloid scars with botulinum toxin.[34]

1. Reconstitute a vial of botulinum toxin according to the manufacturer's instructions for use.
2. Prevention: inject approximately 5U per cm intraleasionally, intradermally at the time of suture removal.[35]
3. Prevention of hypertrophic scarring after epicantoplasty: inject 5U total in 2 injection points (orbicularis oculi muscle and depressor supercilii muscle) (fig. 36).
4. Hypertrophic and keloid scars: treat every 8 weeks with 5U per cm^3.[37] (Note – incobotulinumtoxin recommended for higher frequency than 12-week intervals).

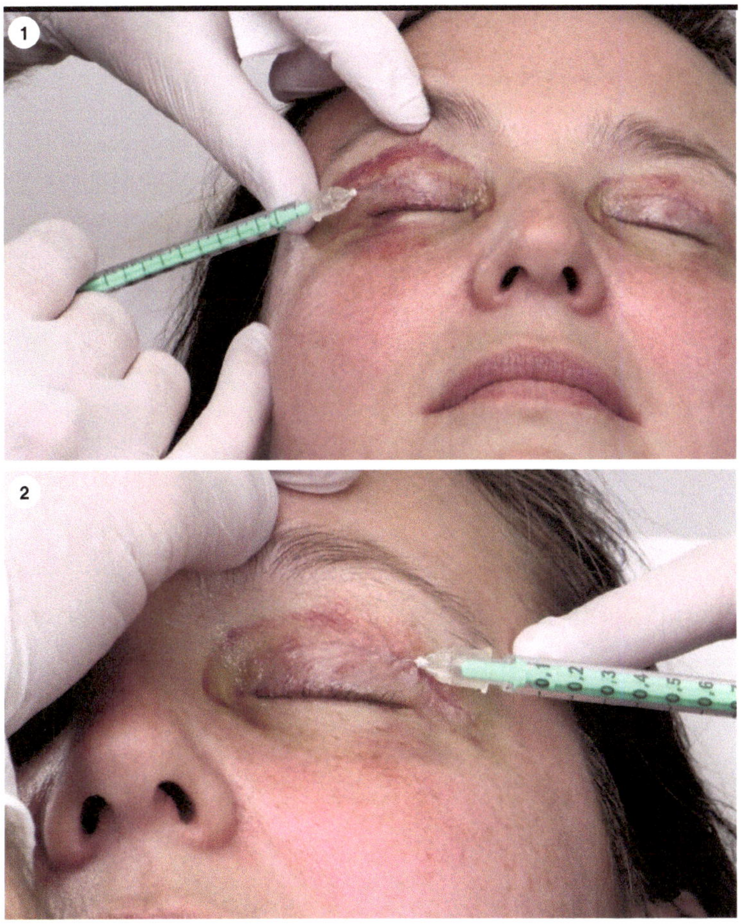

Figure 39
Scars

1 Micro drops of <1 U (<2.5 sU) are injected into the scar.
2 Small retrograde linear threads can also be used for even distribution inside the scar.

For the correction of acne scars, off label mixing of hyaluronic acid and botulinum toxin has been attempted with an automated injection device. Significant reduction of acne scars was shown in this study.[38]

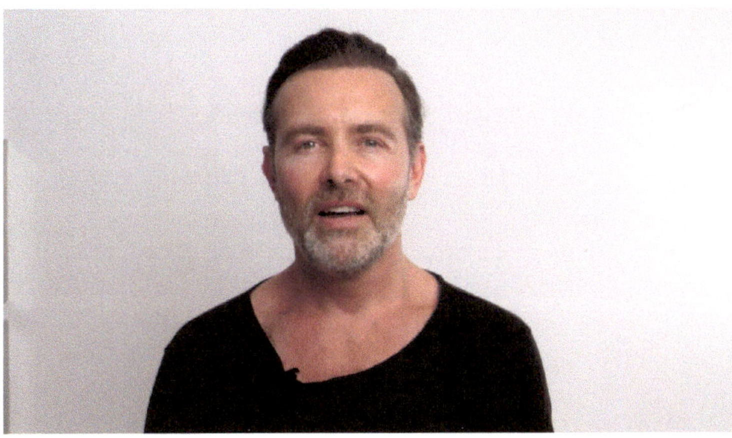

Watch video at http://bit.ly/botulinum-toxin-in-aesthetic-medicine-uma-academy

Video 19
Scars: prevention of hypertrophic scarring after blepharoplasty

The scar was pretreated with topical anesthetic ointment and the sutures were removed. Immediately after suture removal, a total of 4 U (10 sU) was injected on both sides using micro drops or small retrograde linear threads of <1 U (<2.5 sU) per injection point. The dose is conservative to prevent levator ptosis.

skin quality improvement

6.2 Reduction of pore size and sebum production

Skin pores are anatomically skin surface structures corresponding to the outlet of the hair shaft and sebum secretion. Enlarged facial pores can be a matter of cosmetic concern. Enlarged facial pores are primarily treated through addressing associative factors, such as increased sebum production and cutaneous aging. The current treatment modalities for enlarged or dense facial pores include topical retinoids, chemical peels, oral anti-androgens, and laser devices.[39] Novel applications of botulinum toxin injection include intradermal injection in facial skin in low dosages in order to reduce pore size and sebum production.[39-42]

Several theories have been proposed to explain the mechanism of action. First, nicotinic acetylcholine receptors are expressed on sebaceous glands which are able to release acetylcholine. Botulinum toxin effectively blocks the cholinergic signaling and, with that, the sebum production decreases as endogenously produced acetylcholine may alter the production of sebum.[39] Clinically, a decreased activity of the sebaceous glands leads to less seborrhea and thus a reduction in the pore size. Alternatively, the neuromodular effect of botulinum toxin on the musculi arrectores pilorum, causing hairs to stand on end, leads to a decreased sebum excretion, and also relaxation of the musculi arrectores pilorum itself might contribute to a decreased pore size.[45]

Reconstitution of Incobotulinumtoxin and Onabotulinumtoxin is done in 5ml of normal or bacteriostatic saline per 100U for the reduction of pore size and sebum production (off-label). At the area of enlarged pores, 2U (0.1 mL of reconstituted toxin) are injected in an intradermal bleb every 1 cm^2.

Treatment protocol

1. Disinfect the skin
2. Mark the area of enlarged pores and/or excessive sebum production
3. Mark 1x1 cm squares
4. Inject 2U (0.1 mL) of incobotulinumtoxin or abobotulinum toxin intradermally (corresponding with 5U abobotulinumtoxin) per square of 1 cm^2.

Results should be visible after 1-2 weeks and remain for at least four months.
CAVE: make sure you are intradermally as underlying muscles might be affected by deeper injections.

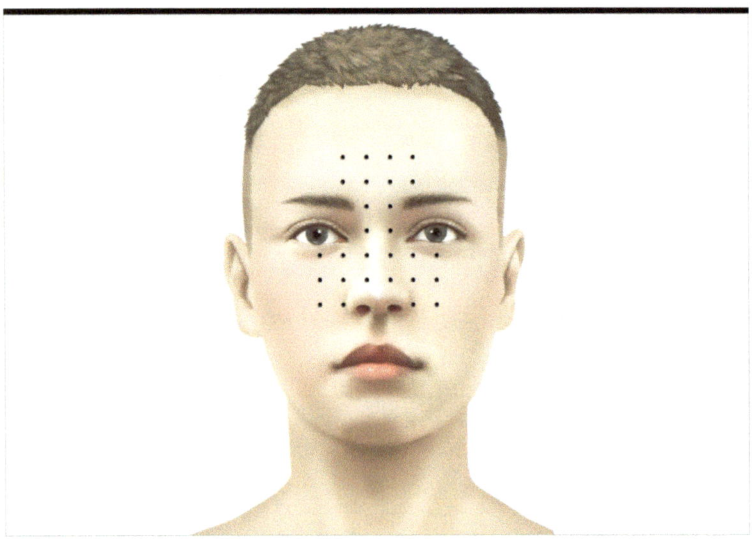

Figure 40
Pores

The area of enlarged pores is injected intradermally every square cm.

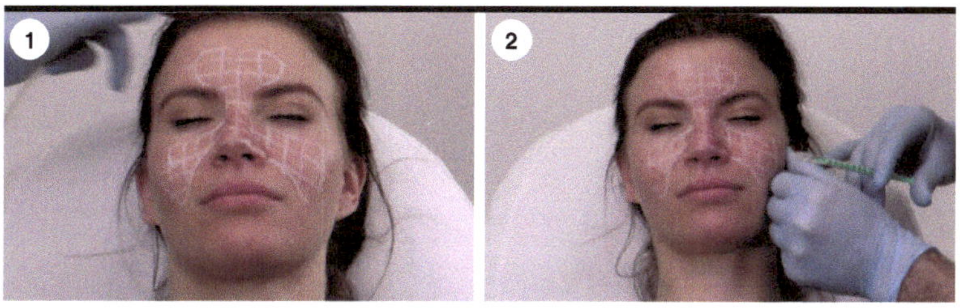

Figure 41
Pores

1 Marking of 1x1 cm squares in the area with enlarged pores.
2 Injection of superficial blebs of diluted botulinum toxin. Note the blanching effect just after injection due to temporary compression of papillary blood vessels, indicating correct intradermal injection.

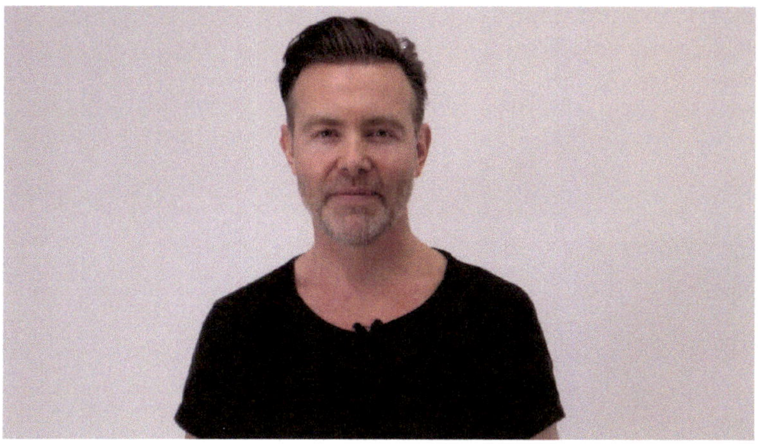

Video 20
Enlarged pores

Watch video at http://bit.ly/botulinum-toxin-in-aesthetic-medicine-uma-academy

6.3 Microtoxin injections for facial lifting

Recent reports showed that facial laxity and skin roughness can be improved, and even facial lifting can be observed using a so-called microbotulinum technique, or Microtoxin technique as we like to call it, where botulinum toxin is injected intradermally.[40-42] These studies also show reduction of pore size and sebum production as described in the previous section.

The treatment approach for this indication is simple. A 1x1 cm grid is drawn on the face (except the eyelids) from the forehead to the cheek and down to the jawline. A total of 100U (250 sU) is reconstituded in normal or bacteriostatic saline. Every cm^2 receives a superficial intradermal bleb of toxin (50U or 125 sU per side, figures 42 and 43).

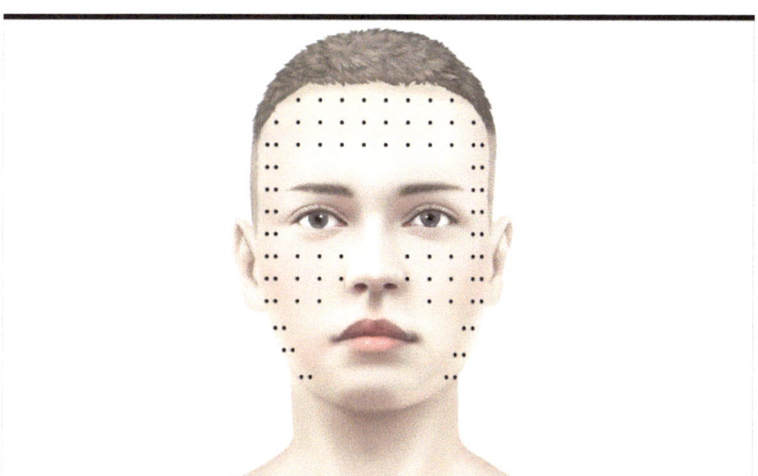

Figure 42
Microtoxin lifting

skin quality improvement

Treatment protocol

1 Disinfect the skin
2 Mark 1x1 cm squares on:
   a Upper forehead (approx. 20 points per side)
   b Temples (approximately 10 points)
   c Cheeks (approximately 40 points)
   d Jawline lateral and inferior (approximately 20 points per side)
3 Count the number of squares (apporox. 100 in total)
4 Reconstitute a vial of toxin according to the following volumes of normal or bacteriostatic saline:[43]
   a 100U IncobotulinumtoxinA (Xeomin / Bocouture) in 6mL[43]
   b 500U AbobotulinumtoxinA (Dysport / Azallure) in 7 mL[44]
   c 100U OnabotulinumtoxinA (Botox / Vistabel) in 5 mL[40]
5 Inject a total of 50 U / 125 sU per hemiface: divide the volume for injection by the number of injection points.
6 Use clinical observation for increasing or decreasing dose per intradermal bleb depending on location and severity of clinical signs.

Results should be visible after 2 weeks and improvements should be visible for approximately 3-4 months.[44]

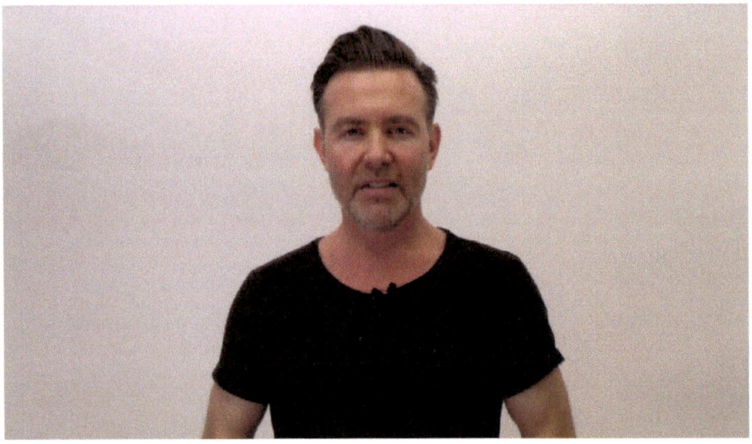

Watch video at http://bit.ly/botulinum-toxin-in-aesthetic-medicine-uma-academy

Video 21
Microtoxin

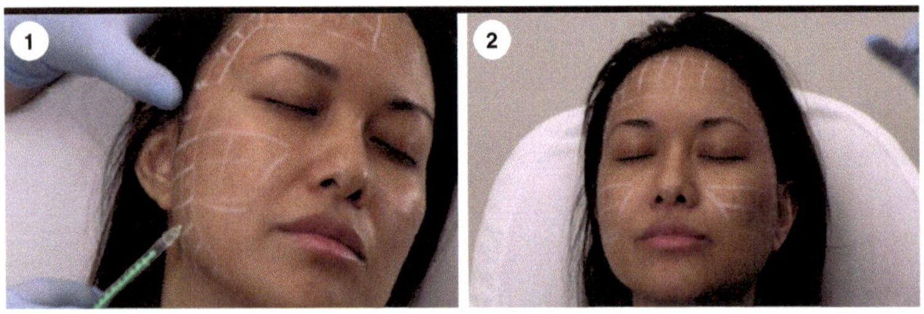

Figure 43
Microtoxin

1 Marking of 1x1 cm squares in the area where skin tightening may give lift to the face.
2 Injection of superficial blebs of diluted botulinum toxin. Note the blanching effect just after injection due to temporary compression of papillary blood vessels, indicating correct intradermal injection.

6.4 Androgenetic alopecia reduction

Androgenetic alopecia (AGA) represents a common aesthetic complaint and is characterized by a progressive miniaturization of the hair follicle.[46] The efficacy and safety of current medical treatment remain limited and include oral finasteride and topical minoxidil.[47] Platelet- Rich Plasma (PRP), Light-Emitting Diode (LED), microneedling, and stem cell injection may also have benefit to the patients suffering from AGA. Intramuscular as well as intradermal injection of Botulinum toxin at the scalp has recently been shown to yield good results in the treatment of AGA.[46-49] The mechanism of action is not yet known, but two main pathways have been proposed. Firstly, relaxation of the muscles of the scalp has been suggested, by reducing the muscular pressure on vessels, allowing a better oxygenation of tissues. For this mechanism of action, intramuscular injection is assumed. Secondly, downregulation of the synthesis of transforming growth factor-β1, which is usually increased by dihydrotestosterone (DHT) has been proposed. For this mechanism of action, intradermal injection is assumed, as DHT has direct effect on the hair follicles.

Approximately 120-150 U / 300-375 sU should be injected evenly in the affected area with approximately 1 U / 2.5 sU per cm^2. Overall results of botulinum toxin injections at the affected sites on the scalp can be improved by prescribing oral finasteride.[46]

Treatment protocol

1. Disinfect the skin
2. Mark 1x1 cm squares on the AGA area (or estimate 1cm distances as marking on thinning hair is not realistic)
3. Count the number of squares
4. Reconstitute a vial of toxin according to the manufacturer's instructions for use
5. Inject 1 U / 2.5 sU per sU per cm^2
6. Total dose should range between 50 and 150 U / 125-375 sU
7. Repeat every 3 months

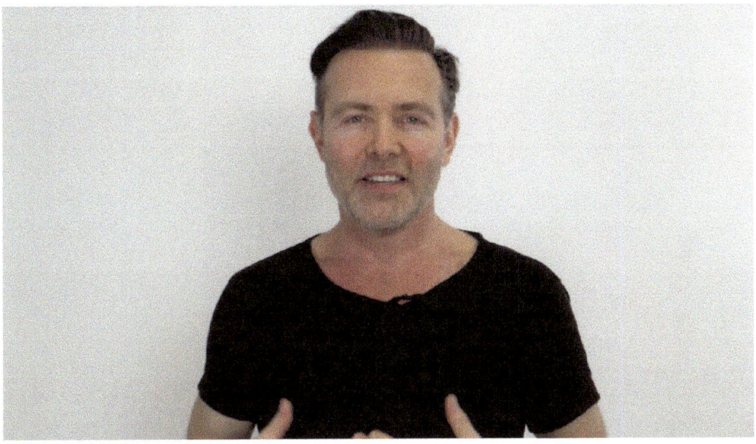

Video 22
Androgenic alopecia

Watch video at http://bit.ly/botulinum-toxin-in-aesthetic-medicine-uma-academy

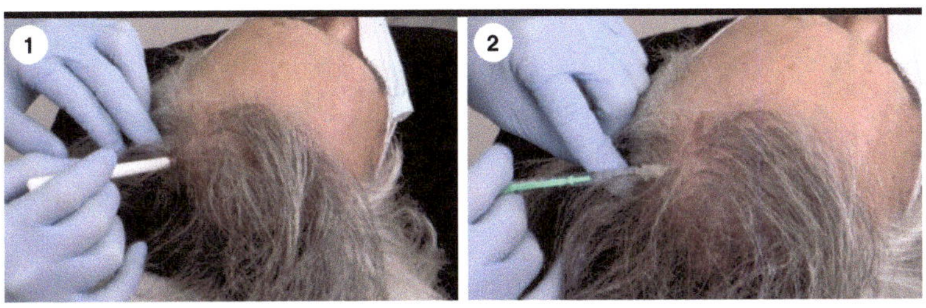

Figure 44
Treatment of androgenic alopecia using botulinum toxin

1. The areas of more severe alopecia (reduced density) are determined.
2. Intradermal blebs of approximately 1 U (2.5 sU) are injected.

6.5 Botulinum toxin for the reduction of flushing, facial erythema and rosacea

Rosacea is a common chronic, inflammatory cutaneous condition that usually affects the convexities of the central face. Symptoms include frequent and prolonged flushing, telangiectasia, papules and pustules, and ocular manifestations, such as burning, stinging sensations and light sensitivities.[50] Even though the etiology is not fully unraveled, rosacea is initiated by genetic and environmental triggers (e.g., spices, alcohol, medicine, temperature). Triggering factors may lead to a dysregulation of the immune system and the cutaneous nervous and vascular system. Various immune related mediators get released, such as mast cells (MC), T helper cells and macrophages. Additionally, a release of vasoactive neuropeptides, by the activation of transient receptor potential vanilloid (TRPV) and transient receptor potential ankyrin (TRPA) on peripheral sensory neurons, lead to the manifestation of rosacea flares.[51,52] Intradermal injection of botulinum toxin may affect both the immune system as well as the hyperactive neurovascular system. Therefore, botulinum toxin has been investigated for the treatment of rosacea.

Vascular influence is the more obvious mechanism of action (MoA). As discussed in chapter 1.2, botulinum toxin type A cleaves SNARE complexes which inhibits the release of acetylcholine (Ach), but it also modulates neuropeptides including vasoactive intestinal peptide (VIP) and calcitonin gene-related peptide (CGRP).[53-56] Ach produces endothelium-dependent vasodilatation through numerous pathways, of which the NO-dependent pathway is the most prominent.[53] VIP and also CGRP causes NO-dependent dilation in vascular beds.[54,59,60] CGRP is a powerful endogenous vasodilator in man which may provoke flushes. Intravenous injections lead to systemic vasodilatation and redistribution of blood flow to the skin.[55-56] Inhibition of these neuromodulators/neuropeptides by botulinum toxin seems a rational MoA to reduce flushes in rosacea. The role of botulinum toxin and the way it affects the immune system is less clear. It is believed that botulinum toxin inhibits MC degranulation, as MC express SNARE complexes.[52] Moreover, the human skin, and more specifically the sweat glands and arterioles in the skin, contain immunoreactive nerve fibers for VIP and VIP receptors. VIP receptors have also been identified on skin MCs.[57-58] Intradermal injection of VIP mediates vasodilation which, in part, is dependent on the release of histamine after MC degranulation.[54]

Botulinum toxin is a promising treatment for rosacea as it not only targets the neurovascular component of rosacea but also the immunologic component. Further studies need to be conducted to optimize treatment protocols in larger sample sizes to confirm efficacy.

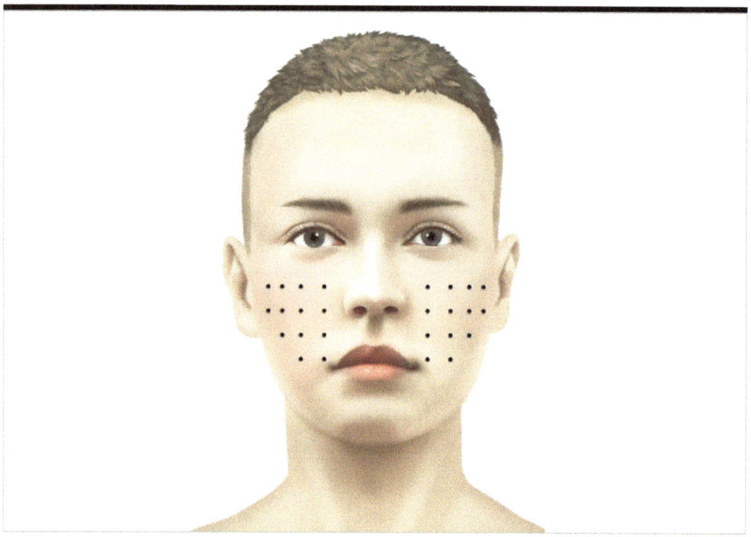

Figure 45
Flushing

Treatment protocol

1 Disinfect the skin
2 Mark 1x1 cm squares on the erythematous lesions of the face
3 Reconstitute a vial of toxin according to the manufacturer's instructions for use, but double the amount of saline: 2.5ml per vial of 50U/1.26ml per vial of 125sU
4 Inject 1 U / 2.5 sU per sU per cm^2
5 Total dose should range between 15 and 50 U / 37.5-125 sU
6 If necessary, repeat after 1 week

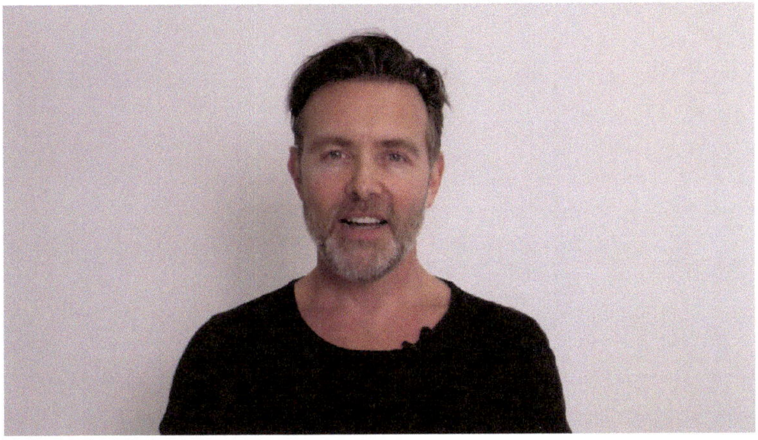

Watch video at http://bit.ly/botulinum-toxin-in-aesthetic-medicine-uma-academy

Video 23
Flushing

Injecting botulinum toxin for reduction of facial erythema (flushing): intradermal blebs of approximately 1 U / 2.5 sU are injected.

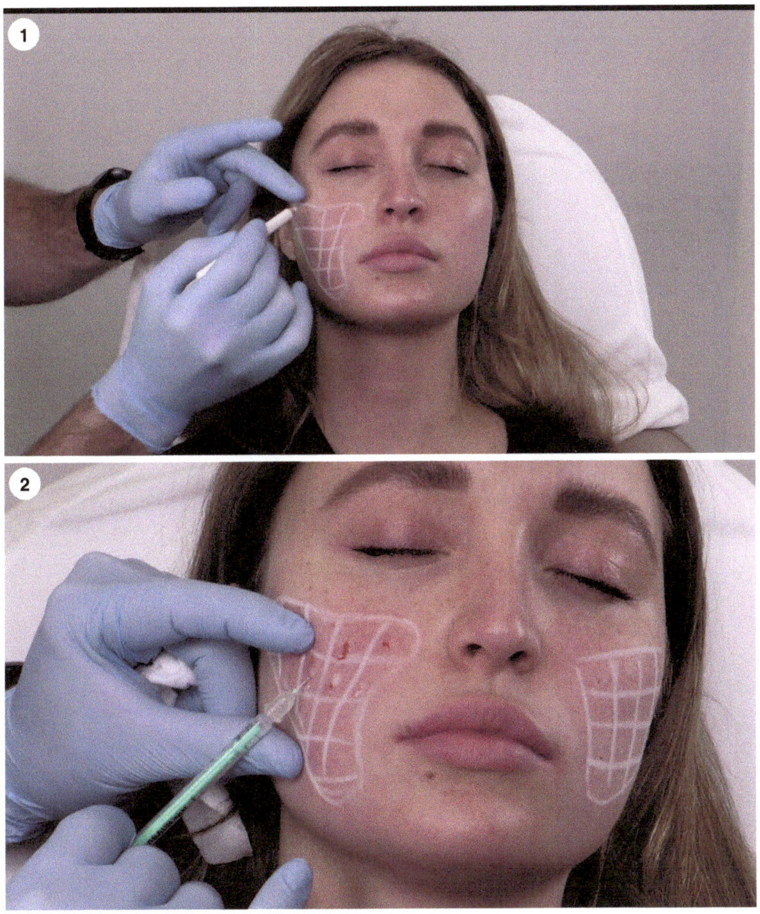

Figure 46
Flushing

1 Marking of the area with 1 x 1 cm squares.
2 Injection of intradermal blebs of approximately 1 U / 2.5 sU.

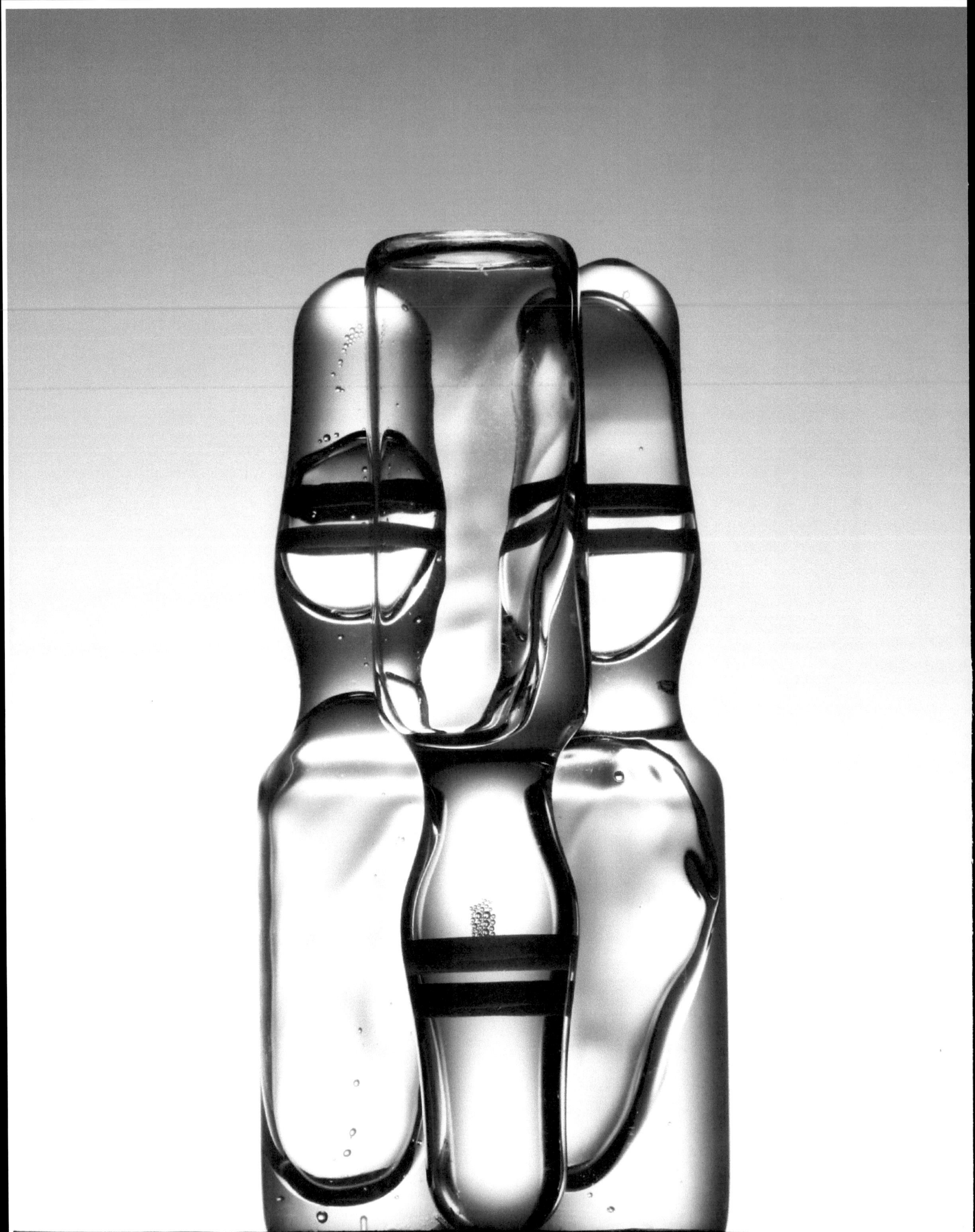

references

1. **Kerner J. Uber das Wurstgift.** *Tübinger Blätter für Naturwissenschaften und Arzney-Kunde* 1817;3:1-25.
2. **Van Ermengem EP.** *Über einen neuen anaeroben Bacillus und seine Beziehung zum Botulismus. Z Hyg Infektionskrankh* 1897;26:1-56 (English version: Van Ermengem EP. A new anaerobic bacillus and its relation to botulism. Rev Infect Dis 1979;1:701-719.
3. **Lamanna C, Amcelroy E, Eklund HW.** *The purification and crystallization of Clostridium Botulinum type A toxin.* Science 1946;103:613-614.
4. **Pidcock FS.** *The emerging role of therapeutic Botulinum toxin in the treatment of cerebral palsy.* J Pediatr 2004;145:S33-S35.
5. **American Society for Aesthetic Plastic Surgery.** *Cosmetic surgery statistics 2015.* Available from: http://www.surgery.org/sites/default/files/Stats2015.pdf. Accessed 12 October, 2016.
6. **Bigalke H, et al.** *Botulinum A toxin: Dysport improvement of biological availability.* Exp Neurol 2001;168:162–170.
7. **Carruthers A, et al.** *The convergence of medicine and neurotoxins: a focus on Botulinum toxin type A and its application in aesthetic medicine—a global, evidence-based Botulinum toxin consensus education initiative: part I: Botulinum toxin in clinical and cosmetic practice.* Dermatol Surg 2013;39:493–509.
8. **Eisele KH, Fink K, Vey M, Taylor HV.** *Studies on the dissociation of Botulinum neurotoxin type A complexes.* Toxicon 2011;57:555–565.
9. **Nestor MS, Ablon GR.** *Comparing the clinical attributes of AbobotulinumtoxinA and OnabotulinumtoxinA utilizing a novel contralateral frontalis model and the frontalis activity measurement standard.* J Drugs Dermatol 2011;10:1148–1157.
10. **Hexsel D, Dal'Forno T, Hexsel C, Do Prado DZ, et al.** *A randomized pilot study comparing the action halos of two commercial preparations of Botulinum toxin type A.* Dermatol Surg 2008;34:52–59.
11. **Allen SB, Goldenburg NA.** *Pain difference associated with injection of AbobotulinumtoxinA reconstituted with preserved saline and preservative-free saline: a prospective, randomized, side-by-side, double-blind study.* Dermatol Surg 2012;38:867–870.
12. **Vadoud-Seyedi J, Simonart T.** *Treatment of axillary hyperhidrosis with Botulinum toxin type A reconstituted in lidocaine or in normal saline: a randomized, side-by-side, double-blind study.* Br J Dermatol 2007;156:986–989.
13. **Imhof M, et al.** *Leitlinie der Deutschen Dermatologischen Gesellschaft Ästhetische Botulinum toxin Therapie.* AWMF Online 2012;(013/077 S1):1-32.
14. **Carruthers J, et al.** *The convergence of medicine and neurotoxins: a focus on Botulinum toxin type A and its application in aesthetic medicine—a global, evidence-based Botulinum toxin consensus education initiative: part II: incorporating Botulinum toxin into aesthetic clinical practice.* Dermatol Surg 2013;39(3 Pt 2):510-525.
15. **Dormston WG, et al.** *Konsensusempfehlungen zur Behandlung mit Onabotulinumtoxin A in der ästhetischen Medizin.* JDDG 2012;(11)1:1-42.
16. **Ascher B, et al.** *International consensus recommendations on the aesthetic usage of Botulinum toxin type A (Speywood Unit) – part I: upper facial wrinkles.* JEADV 2010;24(11):1278-1284.
17. **Wanitphakdeedecha R.** *The effect of Botulinum toxin type A in different dilution on the contraction of fibroblast—In vitro study.* J Cosmet Dermatol. 2019;00:1–9.
18. **Scheinfeld N.** *The use of apraclonidine eyedrops to treat ptosis after the administration of Botulinum toxin to the upper face.* Dermatol Online J 2005;11(1):9.
19. **Wollina U, Konrad H.** *Managing adverse events associated with Botulinum toxin type A: a focus on cosmetic procedures.* Am J Clin Dermatol 2005;6(3):141-150.
20. **Binder WJ, Blitzer A.** *Treatment of migraine headache with Botulinum toxin type A.* Facial Plast Surg Clin N Am 2003;11:465–475.
21. **Ascher B, et al.** *International consensus recommendations on the aesthetic usage of Botulinum toxin type A (Speywood Unit) – part II: wrinkles on the middle and lower face, neck and chest.* JEADV 2010;24(11):1285-1295.
22. **Kim N-H, Chung J-H, Park R-H, et al.** *The use of Botulinum toxin type A in aesthetic mandibular contouring.* Plast Reconstr Surg 2005;115:919–930.
23. **De Sanctis Pecora C., Bussamara Pinheiro M.V., Figueiredo V., Guerra R.** *Evaluation od ONE21 technique with IncobotulinumtoxinA for tratment of forehead wrinkles.* Abstract.
24. **De Sanctis Pecora C.** *Tailored eyebrow shape and positioning using IncobotulinumtoxinA injection in the upper face.* Abstact.
25. **De Sanctis Pecora C., Bussamara Pinheiro M.V.,Ventura Ferreira K., et. Al.** *The ONE21 approach compared with standard 5-point strategy for treating glabellar lines with IncobotulinumtoxinA.* Abstract.
26. **Sohrabi C., Goutos I.** *The use of botulinum toxin in keloid scar management: a literature review.* Scars, Burns & Healing Volume 6: 1–13.
27. **Xiao Z, Zhang F and Lin W.** *Effect of Botulinum Toxin Type A on Transforming Growth Factor b 1 in Fibroblasts Derived from Hypertrophic Scar : A Preliminary Report.*

references

Aesthetic Plast Surg 2010; 34: 424–427.

28. **Xiao Z, Zhang M and Liu Y.** *Botulinum Toxin Type A Inhibits Connective Tissue Growth Factor Expression in Fibroblasts Derived From Hypertrophic Scar.* Aesthetic Plast Surg 2011; 35: 802–807.
29. **Hao RT, Li ZC, Chen X, et al.** *Efficacy and possible mechanisms of Botulinum Toxin type A on hypertrophic scarring.* J Cosmet Dermatol 2018; 17: 340–346.
30. **Xiaoxue W, Xi C and Zhibo X.** *Effects of Botulinum Toxin Type A on Expression of Genes in Keloid Fibroblasts.* Aesthetic Surg J 2014; 34: 154–159.
31. **Zhibo X and Miaobo Z.** *Botulinum toxin type A affects cell cycle distribution of fibroblasts derived from hypertrophic scar.* J Plast Reconstr Aesthetic Surg 2008; 61: 1128–1129.
32. **Jeong HS, Lee BH, Sung HM, et al.** *Effect of Botulinum Toxin Type A on Differentiation of Fibroblasts Derived from Scar Tissue.* Plast Reconstr Surg 2015; 136: 171e–178e.
33. **Bi M., Sun P., Li D., et al.** *Intralesional Injection of Botulinum Toxin Type A Compared with Intralesional Injection of Corticosteroid for the Treatment of Hypertrophic Scar and Keloid: A Systematic Review and Meta-Analysis.* Med Sci Monit, 2019; 25: 2950-2958.
34. **Kasyanju Carrero LM, Ma WW, Liu HF, Yin XF, Zhou BR.** *Botulinum toxin type A for the treatment and prevention of hypertrophic scars and keloids: Updated review.* J Cosmet Dermatol. 2019;18:10–15
35. **Kim SH, Lee SJ, Lee JW, Jeong HS, Suh IS.** *Clinical trial to evaluate the efficacy of botulinum toxin type A injection for reducing scars in patients with forehead laceration: A double-blinded, randomized controlled study.* Medicine (Baltimore) 2019 Aug;98(34):e16952.
36. **Huang RL, Ho CK, Tremp M, Xie Y, Li Q, Zan T.** *Early Postoperative Application of Botulinum Toxin Type A Prevents Hypertrophic Scarring after Epicanthoplasty: A Split-Face, Double-Blind, Randomized Trial.* Plast Reconstr Surg 2019;144(4):835-844.
37. **Shaarawy E, Hegazy RA, Abdel Hay RM.** *Intralesional botulinum toxin type A equally effective and better tolerated than intralesional steroid in the treatment of keloids: a randomized controlled trial.* J Cosmet Dermatol. 2015;14(2):161-166.
38. **Kim JS.** *Topographic computer analysis for acne scar treatment on face accompanying biopsy study after dermal injection of hydrotoxin mixture.* J Cosmet Dermatol 2021 Jan;20(1):75-83.
39. **Sayed KS, Hegazy R, Gawdat HI, Abdel Hay RM, Ahmed MM, Mohammed FN, Allam R, Fahim A.Sayed KS, et al.** *The efficacy of intradermal injections of botulinum toxin in the management of enlarged facial pores and seborrhea: a split face-controlled study.* J Dermatolog Treat. 2020 Jan 3:1-7.
40. **Sapra P, Demay S, Sapra S, Khanna J, Mraud K, Bonadonna J.Sapra P, et al.** *A Single-blind, Split-face, Randomized, Pilot Study Comparing the Effects of Intradermal and Intramuscular Injection of Two Commercially Available Botulinum Toxin A Formulas to Reduce Signs of Facial Aging.* J Clin Aesthet Dermatol. 2017 Feb;10(2):34-44. Epub 2017 Feb 1.
41. **Diaspro A, Calvisi L, Manzoni V, Sito G.Diaspro A, et al.** *Microbotulinum: A Quantitative Evaluation of Aesthetic Skin Improvement in 62 Patients.* Plast Reconstr Surg. 2020 Nov;146(5):987-994.
42. **Park JY, Cho SI, Hur K, Lee DH.Park JY, et al.** *Intradermal Microdroplet Injection of Diluted Incobotulinumtoxin-A for Sebum Control, Face Lifting, and Pore Size Improvement.* J Drugs Dermatol. 2021 Jan 1;20(1):49-54. doi: 10.36849/JDD.5616.
43. **Wanitphakdeedecha R, Nokdhes YN, Patthamalai P, Yan C, Techapichetvanich T, Phothong W, Eimpunth S, Manuskiatti W.** Dermatol Ther. 2020 Nov;33(6):e13944.
44. **Wanitphakdeedecha R, Yan C, Apinuntham C, Rojanavanich V, Cembrano KAG, Eimpunth S, Manuskiatti W.** *Intradermal Micro-Dosing of AbobotulinumtoxinA for Face-Lifting: How Long Does It Last?* Dermatol Ther (Heidelb). 2020 Aug;10(4):779-789.
45. **Rose AE, Goldberg DJ.** *Safety and efficacy of intradermal injection of botulinum toxin for the treatment of oily skin.* Dermatol Surg. 2013;39:443–448.
46. **Zhou Y, Yu S, Zhao J, Feng X, Zhang M, Zhao Z.** *Effectiveness and Safety of Botulinum Toxin Type A in the Treatment of Androgenetic Alopecia.* Biomed Res Int. 2020 Aug 4;2020:1501893.
47. **Carloni R, Pechevy L, Postel F, Zielinski M, Gandolfi S.J** *Is there a therapeutic effect of botulinum toxin on scalp alopecia? Physiopathology and reported cases: A systematic review of the literature.* Plast Reconstr Aesthet Surg. 2020 Dec;73(12):2210-2216. doi: 10.1016/j.bjps.2020.05.035. Epub 2020 May 22.
48. **Shon U, Kim MH, Lee DY, Kim SH, Park BC.** *The effect of intradermal botulinum toxin on androgenetic alopecia and its possible mechanism.* J Am Acad Dermatol. 2020 Dec;83(6):1838-1839.
49. **Singh S, Neema S, Vasudevan B.J** Cutan Aesthet Surg. *A Pilot Study to Evaluate Effectiveness of Botulinum Toxin in Treatment of Androgenetic Alopecia in Males.* 2017 Jul-Sep;10(3):163-167.
50. **Gallo R.L.,Granstein R.D., Kang S., et. al.** *Standard*

classification and pathophysiology of rosacea: The 2017 update by the National Rosacea Society Expert Committee. J Am Acad Dermatol. 2018. PMID: 29089180 Review.

51. **Sulk M., Seeliger S., Aubert J., et. Al.** *Distribution and Expression of Non-Neuronal Transient Receptor Potential (TRPV) Ion Channels in Rosacea.* J Invest Dermatol. 2012 Apr;132(4):1253-62.
52. **Choi J.E., Werbel T., Wang Z., et. Al.** *Botulinum toxin blocks mast cells and prevents rosacea like Inflammation.* J Dermatol Sci. 2019 Jan;93(1):58-64.
53. **Holowatz L.A, Thompson C.S., Minson C.T., Kenney W.L.** *Mechanisms of acetylcholine mediated vasodilatation in young and aged human skin.* J. Physiol. 2005 Mar;(563):965–73.
54. **Wilkins B.W., Chung L.H., Tublitz N.J, et. Al.** *Mechanisms of vasoactive intestinal peptide mediated vasodilation in human skin.* J. Appl. Physiol. 2004 Oct 4;(97):1291–98.
55. **Raynaud A., Cohen R., Modigliani E.** *Calcitonin gene-related peptide (CGRP).* Presse Med. 1994 Feb 5;23(4):171-5. (in French).
56. **Meng J., Wang J., Lawrence G.,Dolly D.O.** *Synaptobrevin I mediates exocytosis of CGRP from sensory neurons and inhibition by botulinum toxins reflects their anti-nociceptive potential.* J. Cell. Sci. 2007 Aug;(120):2864–2874.
57. **Jansen-Olesen I., Ottosson A., Cantera L., et. Al.** *Role of endothelium and nitric oxide in histamine-induced responses in human cranial arteries and detection of mRNA encoding H1- and H2-receptors by RT-PCR.* Br J Pharmacol. 1997 121: 41–48.
58. **Groneberg D.A., Welker P., Fischer T.C., et. Al.** *Down-regulation of vasoactive intestinal polypeptide receptor expression in atopic dermatitis.* J Allergy Clin Immunol. 2003 111: 1099–1105.
59. **Bloom B.S., Payongayong L., Mourin A., Goldber D.J.** *Impact of Intradermal AbobotulinumtoxinA on Facial Erythema of Rosacea.* Dermatol Surg 2015;41:S9–S16
60. **Park K.Y., Hyun M.Y., Jeong S.Y., et. Al.** *Botulinum Toxin for the Treatment of Refractory Erythema and Flushing of Rosacea.* Dermatology 2015;230:299–301.
61. **Kerscher M, Fabi S, Fischer T, et al.** *IncobotulinumtoxinA Demonstrates Safety and Prolonged Duration of Effect in a Dose-Ranging Study for Glabellar Lines.* J Drugs Dermatol. 2020;19(10)
62. **Keller JE.** *Recovery from botulinum neurotoxin poisoning in vivo.* Neuroscience. 2006;139(2):629-37.
63. **Pellett S, Bradshaw M, Tepp WH, et al.** *The light chain defines the duration of action of botulinum toxin serotype A subtypes.* mBio. 2018;9(2):e00089-18.
64. **Cheng J, Chung HJ, Friedland M, Hsu SH.** *Botulinum Toxin Injections for Leg Contouring in East Asians.* Dermatol Surg. 2020 Oct;46 Suppl 1:S62-S70.

about the author

Jani van Loghem, MD PhD

All our stories begin long before we were born. Jani van Loghem's starts with his grandparents. As pioneering immunologists, the pair travelled the world establishing a nascent medical field, training fellow doctors and changing lives. Their legacy also inspired a young Jani to complete medical school - where he naturally vowed to stay out of the unethical world of commercial medicine.

It was while working as a junior doctor in the general surgery department, that he first encountered the world of injectables - and it was love at first sight. The positivity one brought to patients' lives. The lack of superiors to boss one around. Jani began diving into the literature, taking workshops and going to aesthetic conferences. And the more he learned, the more he realised he needed to learn. Just like his grandparents before him, Jani was at the forefront of a new medical speciality. Merely running a successful clinic was not enough – he had the chance to be part of its development.

Jani's relentless passion for aesthetic medicine was key to the Netherlands being the first country in the world to recognise it as a two year specialism. Since then, his work has taken him around the world, sharing his experience and understanding with other professionals so that everyone can raise their game. Asked what advice he would have for his younger self today, Jani replies, "Follow your heart."

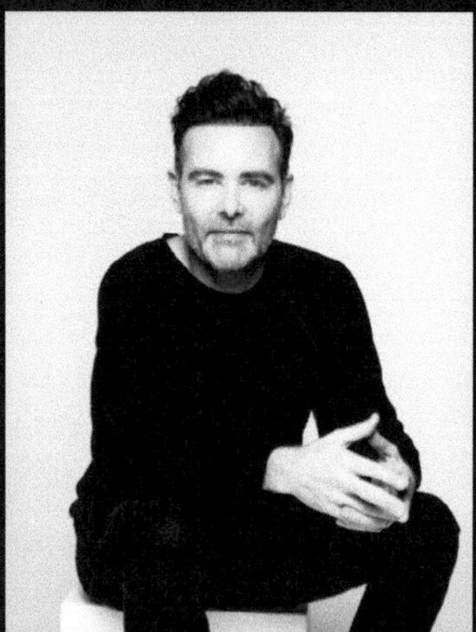

our curriculum

Our curriculum of book publications, webinars, discourses and hands-on training is created by the same team who developed The Netherlands' medical specialty of aesthetic medicine. Tailor-made for the digital age, our courses combine a solid theoretical background with clinical training, with unprecedented access to the expertise of some of the industry's top practitioners.

toxins

toxin essentials

advanced toxin techniques

soft tissue fillers

filler essentials

advanced filler techniques

complication prevention & management

attractiveness

female beauty

male attractiveness

intimate areas

aesthetic surgery

facial surgery

body contouring

oculoplastics

aesthetic skin therapy

energy based devices

chemical peels

needling and skin boosters

For more information visit our website **www.uma-institute.com** and get acces to a wide range of courses, events, webinars, books and online learning materials.

your notes

index